CASE STUDIES
FOR INTERPRETING THE
MMPI-A

CASE STUDIES
FOR INTERPRETING THE
MMPI-A

Yossef S. Ben–Porath
and
Daniel L. Davis

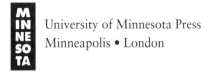

University of Minnesota Press
Minneapolis • London

"MMPI," "MMPI-2," "MMPI-A," and "Minnesota Multiphasic Personality Inventory," "Minnesota Multiphasic Personality Inventory-2," and Minnesota Multiphasic Personality Inventory-Adolescent" are trademarks owned by the University of Minnesota.

Published by the University of Minnesota Press
111 Third Avenue South, Suite 290
Minneapolis, MN 55401-2520

CIP data available. ISBN 0-8166-2729-0

CONTENTS

PART 1. MMPI-A BACKGROUND

PART 2. MMPI-A CASES

FOREWORD

For a psychological assessment instrument to become a standard in its field it must possess a number of features or properties: It must have content relevance and address qualities that are important to clinical decision-making, it must be psychometrically sound, that is, possess measures that have reliability, and, finally, it must hold the promise of predicting that which it is supposed to predict in an effective manner. This last attribute refers both to external validation and clinical utility.

Assessing the validity of a psychological test is often thought to involve only statistical coefficients that tie test indices to behavior. However, much more is required, ultimately involving the careful documentation of how the instrument performs in complex assessment tasks. This requirement, often ignored or minimized in the evaluation of any psychological test, includes the development of clinical lore, an important element of any psychological test that emerges when it is applied in real-world settings. If a psychological test is to be a major instrument in a field, it must have an expanding empirical research base and must also be blessed with an extensive base of successful application. "Case Studies for Interpreting the MMPI-A" by Yossef S. Ben-Porath and Daniel L. Davis provides such a landmark for the Minnesota Multiphasic Personality Inventory for Adolescents (MMPI-A).

This book represents a substantial effort to explore broadly how the MMPI-A is used in describing and predicting the behavior of adolescents who are experiencing psychological problems. Although the authors have taken a "case-oriented" approach, the book is more than a collection of clinical cases. It is an instructional resource for professionals working with adolescents and for child-clinical graduate students that provides clear interpretive guidelines and an effective strategy for understanding adolescents through the use of the MMPI-A. Although this book will be of most value to those who have some experience in MMPI interpretation with adolescents, it should prove useful to neophytes as well since it provides sufficient background in the use of the MMPI instruments with adolescents.

The heart of this casebook is the rich clinical material that the authors have gleaned from many clinical contexts. The cases represent a very broad range of problems from typical clinical settings. Each of the 16 cases is presented in a standard fashion, in which all the important elements of a good case study are included.

What is most critical is the authors' provision of very detailed case records — personal history and problem manifestation — which make very clear what problems are being assessed. The authors also provide a skillful interpretive analysis of the adolescent's MMPI-A scores. These profile interpretations are integrated nicely into the case-history information to reflect the diagnostic formulation and treatment recommendations for each case. Finally, the authors also provide follow-up or outcome

FOREWORD

information to enable the reader to determine what happened with each of the adolescents described in the book.

The authors of this casebook on the MMPI-A, Yossef S. Ben-Porath and Daniel L. Davis, are unusually well suited for the task of developing an effective casebook. Professor Ben-Porath was actively involved in the research on and development of the MMPI-A, and is very knowledgeable about the psychometric factors underlying the test. He has maintained a very productive research program on the MMPI instruments in which the MMPI-A has been a major focus. Moreover, he has been extensively involved in teaching the MMPI-A in professional workshops for many years and has a clear understanding of what beginning students need to know about the MMPI-A to employ it effectively. His co-author, Daniel L. Davis, is an expert in the area of juvenile delinquency and has been involved in the rehabilitation of youth in various correctional programs for many years. Both authors have a very substantial clinical background in assessing adolescent clients. Their case selection and case descriptions of the adolescents included in this volume show great sensitivity regarding the issues facing clinicians whose task it is to assess adolescent clients.

James N. Butcher
University of Minnesota

PREFACE

This book is designed to serve as an instructional and general reference resource for clinicians and clinicians–in–training who wish to use the recently published adolescent version of the MMPI, the MMPI–A. It consists of two parts, the first providing background information on the instrument, the second, presenting the cases of 16 adolescents who completed the MMPI–A in a variety of clinical settings.

In writing this book we assumed that the reader has already mastered the basic reference materials related to the MMPI–A. As with any psychological test, it is recommended that those who use the MMPI–A be thoroughly familiar with the psychometric and other information provided in the test manual. Part 1 begins with the introduction in which we discuss a number of sources containing additional information that should prove helpful to those interpreting the MMPI–A. A strategy for interpreting the MMPI–A is provided in the next chapter. We have found this strategy helpful in a variety of clinical and referral contexts and have used it in interpreting the cases presented in this volume.

Part 2 provides the 16 cases we have chosen to illustrate various issues and approaches to MMPI–A interpretation. The cases come from a broad range of settings and cover a wide variety of referral issues. For each case we provide the available background information (with masking of identifying information), clinical observations of the youngster, an annotated interpretation, and outcome information to the extent that it was available. Our annotated interpretations provide a detailed analysis of each profile and an account of how we derived our interpretations from the available information. In the final chapter we provide concluding remarks concerning the cases and the contribution of the MMPI-A in assessing adolescent functioning and behavior.

Collection of the cases and the information contained in this volume was facilitated substantially by a number of individuals who worked with us on this project. Yossef Ben–Porath wishes to acknowledge the assistance of several students who worked with him at Kent State University: Danielle Darkangelo, Eileen McCully, Jennifer Oldenberg, and Lebron Rankins. At the time we collected these cases, Daniel Davis served as the Clinical Director of the Buckeye Ranch in Grove City, Ohio, the source for a number of cases included in this volume. Presently Dr. Davis is affiliated with the Ohio Department of Rehabilitation and Corrections. Acknowledgment is gratefully given to Ms. Heidi Stelzig for her invaluable assistance to Dr. Davis. Without her involvement in the selection, initial drafting, and editing of the case studies, his participation and contributions to this effort would not have been possible.

We wish to express our appreciation and gratitude to Beverly Kaemmer, of the University of Minnesota Press, for her editorial input and guidance and her long–standing support of our research efforts with the MMPI–A. We thank Richard Rumer for his helpful comments as a reviewer of our manuscript. We also wish to thank National Computer Systems

PREFACE

(NCS) and Troy Juliar for the provision of software used to produce the MMPI–A profiles included in this volume.

Last, but not least, we wish to acknowledge our appreciation and regard for the 16 youngsters whose MMPI–A profiles we interpret in this book. We hope that our efforts and theirs will serve to illustrate how the MMPI–A can be used to identify the needs and strengths of adolescents evaluated in various clinical settings.

Yossef S. Ben–Porath and Daniel L. Davis
June 1996
Kent, Ohio

PART

1

MMPI-A
BACKGROUND

INTRODUCTION

The Minnesota Multiphasic Personality Inventory–Adolescent (MMPI–A; Butcher, Graham, Williams, Archer, Tellegen, Ben–Porath, & Kaemmer, 1992) is an adaptation of the original MMPI (Hathaway & McKinley, 1943) for use with adolescents. Although the MMPI was developed for use with adults, shortly after its publication researchers and clinicians began to administer the test to teen-agers (e.g., Capwell, 1945a; 1945b). In spite of several obvious shortcomings (e.g., items related to adolescent experiences, such as school, were worded in the past tense; adolescents were absent from the original MMPI normative sample), the test was incorporated into adolescent assessment procedures, and research indicated that it could provide useful descriptive and predictive information on this population (Hathaway & Monachesi, 1953).

Much of what was known about using the original MMPI with adolescents came from two landmark studies, the first by Hathaway and Monachesi (1953, 1957, 1963) the second by Marks, Seeman, and Haller (1974). Starke Hathaway, one of the developers of the MMPI, and Elio Monachesi, a sociologist who collaborated with Hathaway in his adolescent MMPI research, embarked upon an ambitious longitudinal study in which they tested over 15,000 adolescents with the MMPI in the early and mid-1950s and followed these teens' development for a period of 15 years. They were interested in determining whether certain personality characteristics, as mea-sured by the MMPI, might place an adolescent at increased or decreased risk for later engaging in juvenile delinquent behavior.

Hathaway and Monachesi found that several MMPI scales were predictive of later likelihood of juvenile delinquency. Based upon their findings, they divided the MMPI clinical scales into two classes, *excitatory* and *inhibitory*. The excitatory scales, 4, 6, 8, and 9, were correlated positively with subsequent tendencies toward delinquent, aggressive behavior. The inhibitory scales, 2, 3, 5, 7, and 0, were correlated negatively with the same outcome variables. Thus, adolescents with elevated scores on the excitatory scales were viewed as being at increased risk for delinquency whereas those youth with elevated scores on the inhibitory scales were viewed as being at decreased risk for such problems.

To date, Hathaway and Monachesi's study remains unparalleled in its scope and comprehensiveness. However, as the MMPI began to be used increasingly with adolescents in clinical settings, a need arose for research to guide clinicians in interpreting the MMPI profiles of teen-agers who were administered the test in these facilities. This need was addressed by the work of Marks, Seeman, and Haller who, in 1974, published a codebook for interpreting adolescents' MMPI profiles.

Marks et al.'s (1974) effort to identify empirical correlates for adolescent MMPI profiles followed in the tradition of similar studies that had been conducted previously with adult MMPI profiles. Shortly after the

INTRODUCTION

development of the MMPI, researchers and clinicians began to discover that certain patterns of scores on the profile were related consistently to particular personality traits, behavioral tendencies, and symptoms of psychopathology. Following Meehl's (1954) demonstration of the superiority of empirically based assessment over clinical assessment, and his subsequent call for the development of "cookbooks" to guide clinicians in generating empirically based interpretations of the MMPI, several such systems were developed in the 1960s for use with adult MMPI profiles. Marks et al.'s (1974) study represented an extension of these efforts to adolescent MMPI profiles.

Marks at al. (1974) collected extensive data on 834 adolescents who had completed the MMPI and who had been seen for several therapy sessions. The data they collected included self–ratings, ratings by subjects' therapists, and information obtained from the adolescents' clinical records. Marks et al. classified their subjects according to the two highest scales in their profile and assigned nearly every case a two–point code type. Marks et al. (1974) conducted various statistical analyses to identify empirical correlates (external variables that are correlated with membership in a given code type) for those two–point code types for which they had at least ten subjects.

Marks et al. (1974) provided a rich and detailed set of empirically based descriptors for use in interpreting adolescents' MMPI profiles. In addition, these authors published a set of adolescent–specific norms that had been reported previously in Volume I of *An MMPI Handbook* (Dahlstrom, Welsh, & Dahlstrom, 1972). These norms were stratified into a number of age groups and were recommended for use along with the original adult norms when interpreting adolescents' MMPI profiles.

The publication and use of adolescent–specific norms represented a sharp deviation from prior applications of the MMPI with adolescents. Hathaway and Monachesi (1953) had earlier argued against this practice based on the premise

that normative differences between adults and adolescents stemmed from clinically meaningful aspects of adolescence, and that to use adolescent norms would have the effect of obscuring these differences and obfuscating adolescent assessment. However, research and clinical practice indicated that scoring their MMPI profiles based on adult norms often produced artificially high scores for adolescents.

With the availability of empirical descriptors based upon research with adolescent MMPI profiles and adolescent–specific norms for scoring these protocols, use of the MMPI with adolescents began to increase. As described by Archer (1987), the MMPI was used with increasing frequency with adolescents in a variety of clinical and nonclinical settings. However, debates continued regarding the most appropriate method for interpreting adolescents' MMPI profiles.

Butcher and Williams (1992) summarized the various approaches that had been developed for interpreting adolescent MMPI profiles. These included, the *Adult Interpretive Approach*, in which adult norms and correlates were used to interpret adolescents' MMPI profiles, the *Adolescent Interpretive Approach*, in which, following the work of Marks et al. (1974), adolescents' MMPI profiles were scored using adolescent norms and interpretations were based on adolescent correlates, the *Mixed Interpretive Approach*, in which adolescents' profiles were scored using adolescent norms and interpreted on the basis of adult correlates, the *Combined Interpretive Approach*, a method suggested by Archer (1987), in which adolescent profiles were generated with adolescent norms and interpreted on the basis of descriptors from both the adult and adolescent research literature.

Regardless of which method of scoring and interpretation was used, it had become increasingly clear by the late 1970s that problems in using the MMPI with adolescents were not limited to debates over which norms and descriptors to use. Questions were raised increasingly about the appropriateness of the adult and adolescent norms, since both normative samples were based on data collected primarily during the 1940s and 1950s.

In addition to concerns regarding norms, questions were raised about the appropriateness of the MMPI item pool for use with adolescents. Butcher and Williams (1992) summarized these concerns, which included the use of out–of–date language, the inappropriateness for most younger adolescents of items dealing with sexual behavior, the limited applicability of the item pool to adolescent–specific concerns, and the length of the MMPI booklet, particularly in light of the fact that only 383 of the 550 items in the MMPI were scored on routinely interpreted scales.

As early as the late 1960s experts in MMPI research and interpretation began increasingly to raise concerns about the adequacy of the MMPI norms and item pool for use with adults as well as with adolescents. As a result, in 1982 the University of Minnesota Press, publisher of the MMPI, appointed a committee of scholars who were charged with the mission of updating the instrument. The committee was composed of James N. Butcher, of the University of Minnesota, W. Grant Dahlstrom, of the University of North Carolina, John R. Graham, of Kent State University, Auke Tellegen, of the University of Minnesota, and Beverly Kaemmer, of the University of Minnesota Press.

The MMPI Restandardization Committee launched a decade–long project that culminated in the publication in 1989 of an updated version of the MMPI for use with adults, the MMPI–2 (Butcher, Dahlstrom, Graham, Tellegen, & Kaemmer, 1989). Although focussing most of its efforts initially on updating the inventory for use with adults, the committee, in collaboration with Carolyn L. Williams, of the University of Minnesota and Robert P. Archer, of Eastern Virginia University, collected data to explore the feasibility of developing a separate, adolescent–specific version of the instrument. These efforts involved the development of an experimental adolescent version of the MMPI and the collection of two large data sets, one normative, the other clinical. The Press appointed the MMPI Adolescent Project Committee, composed of James N. Butcher, Robert P. Archer, Auke Tellegen, and Beverly Kaemmer to develop a separate instrument for adolescents, which was accomplished with the publication of the MMPI-A in 1992.

DEVELOPMENT OF THE MMPI–A

The first step in constructing the MMPI–A was the development of an experimental form that was used to collect data for the project. This form, called the MMPI–TX, included all 550 original MMPI items and 154 new, experimental items. Some of the new items were also included in the MMPI–AX, the experimental form used to develop the MMPI–2, whereas others were written specifically to address adolescent–relevant issues and were exclusive to the MMPI–TX. Examples of some adolescent–specific items are:

- My parents do not understand me very well.
- I am often upset by things that happen at school.
- I want to go to college.

Two very large samples of adolescents were tested with the MMPI–TX. The normative sample was collected in high schools throughout the United States, with data collected from over 2,000 students. In addition to the MMPI–TX, all of these youngsters completed a detailed biographical information form and a recent life events questionnaire. Subjects who produced invalid profiles were deleted from the sample which was then stratified to come as close as possible to providing a representative sampling of the racial composition of the current adolescent population of the United States. This resulted in a final sample composed of 1,620 adolescents (815 girls and 805 boys). The MMPI-A manual (Butcher et al., 1992) provides highly detailed information regarding the composition of the normative sample.

Using these normative data, the authors developed new adolescent–specific norms for the MMPI–A. In the tradition of the original MMPI, separate norms were developed for adolescent boys and girls. Standard scores were developed for the validity and clinical scales, some of which were slightly modified versions of the original MMPI scales. In addition, new validity, content, and supplementary scales were normed based upon the responses of this sample.

A second sample, a large group of over 800 adolescents tested with the MMPI–TX in various clinical settings, was collected by Williams and Butcher (1989). These data were crucial in the development of the MMPI–A content scales (Williams, Butcher, Ben–Porath, & Graham, 1992) and the new MMPI–A substance-use scales (Weed, Butcher, & Williams, 1994).

In addition to self–completed data from the MMPI–TX, the biographical information form, and the recent life events questionnaires, a broad range of extra–test data were obtained on these subjects. A standardized, comprehensive record review was conducted to extract information systematically and reliably from the treatment records of all of the youngsters in this sample. In addition, for large subsamples of the clinical sample, one parent completed the Child Behavior Checklist (CBCL, Achenbach & Edelbrock, 1983) and treatment staff completed the Devereux Adolescent Behavior Rating Scales (DAB). Based on data collected for this project, new scales were developed for the DAB by Ben–Porath, Williams, and Uchiyama (1989). These extra–test data were used to provide initial information regarding the validity of the MMPI–A clinical and content scales.

A detailed description of the development of the MMPI–A is beyond the scope of this book. For further information, the reader is referred to the MMPI–A manual (Butcher et al., 1992) and to the following reference sources containing information on the MMPI–A (Archer, 1992; Butcher & Williams, 1992; Graham, 1993) and the

book by Williams at al. (1992) describing the development of the MMPI–A Content Scales.

OVERVIEW OF THE MMPI–A

The MMPI–A is a 478–item self–report inventory designed for use with adolescents ranging in age from 14[1] to 18. The test is administered either in booklet form, where the adolescent marks an answer sheet "True" or "False" (or enters no response) in response to each of the test items, or it may be administered by computer, where the adolescent responds to the test items that are presented on a monitor by pressing the appropriate keys for the responses "True," "False," or "Cannot Say." The responses are then scored on scales that are categorized as validity, clinical, content, or supplementary.

Following is a brief overview of the MMPI–A scales. The reader is referred to the previously cited MMPI–A reference sources for more detailed descriptions of the development and interpretation of these scales.

Validity Scales

One of the hallmarks of the MMPI tests (MMPI, MMPI–2, and MMPI–A) is a set of scales that provide the test–interpreter with detailed information regarding the quality of the test responses that form the basis of the interpretation. When they developed the MMPI, Hathaway and McKinley (1943) believed that by constructing empirically keyed scales they would be able to minimize (but not eliminate) the possibility that the test taker would (intentionally or unintentionally) provide misleading information when responding to the test items. Because they knew that even empirically keyed scales remain susceptible to distorting response styles, they developed scales to identify the occurrence of such response styles, thereby alerting the interpreter to the particular problems that may have been introduced. This tradition has been continued and expanded with the MMPI–A, which contains six validity scales.

We describe the validity scales and their interpretation in somewhat more detail than we do the other scales because we think it very important to have an accurate picture of a youngster's test–taking approach. Although profile validity is always a matter of concern for users of the MMPI instruments, when working with adolescents, who often are less than enthusiastic about completing self–report instruments, a thorough analysis of a teen's approach to the test is vital to the validity of the interpretation.

Cannot Say

Cannot Say (CNS) is not a scale in the traditional sense of a psychometric instrument. It is simply a count of the number of items that the adolescent has left unanswered, or has answered both "True" and "False." Too many unanswered items can result in artificially low scores on the remaining scales of the profile (including all of the other validity scales). In general, protocols with more than 30 omitted items are considered invalid.[2] However, if most of the omissions occur after item 350, it is possible to interpret the clinical scales and validity scales L, F_1, and K, because all of the items for these scales appear within the first 350 items of the MMPI–A booklet.

With the advent of computerized scoring, it is possible to take the interpretation of Cannot Say several steps further. Most scoring systems now routinely provide a list of omitted items. When a substantial number of items has been omitted, examination of their content may reveal areas that the youngster is particularly reluctant to address and may suggest further inquiry into the reasons for this hesitancy. In addition, some scoring systems now report the percentage of items answered for each scale. This provides the interpreter with further information regarding content areas that have been avoided as well as direct information regarding which scales are likely affected, and to what extent, by a given set of omitted items.

Lie

The Lie scale (L) was developed by Hathaway and McKinley to identify individuals who attempt to portray themselves as unrealistically virtuous. It is made up of 14 items, all keyed "False." An adolescent who produces a T score greater than 65 on this scale may be attempting to portray her- or himself in an overly favorable light. The greater the elevation, the greater the likelihood that such a response style has occurred.

In interpreting this scale clinicians need to consider two alternative explanations for elevated scores. First, adolescents who come from very traditional backgrounds tend to produce higher than average scores on this scale. Second, because all of the items on this scale are keyed "False," an adolescent who responds "False" indiscriminantly to many of the MMPI–A items will score higher than average on this scale, and an adolescent who responds "True" indiscriminantly to many of the test items will score lower than average on this scale. These two response styles are termed, respectively, *Nay-Saying* and *Yea-Saying*. Both can be detected with the aid of the new validity scale TRIN described below.

The Infrequency Scales

The original MMPI contained an infrequency scale, F, that was composed of 64 items that were rarely endorsed in the keyed direction by subjects in the original normative sample. This was one of the more problematic scales in working with adolescents because youngsters would routinely score very high on this scale when their scores were plotted on adult norms. An analysis of data from the MMPI–A normative sample revealed that many of the original F items are endorsed rather frequently by adolescents. Consequently, a new F scale was developed. Any item endorsed by 20% or fewer of both the girls and the boys in the MMPI-A normative sample was included on this scale.

The MMPI–A F scale contains 66 items that are spread throughout the test booklet. It is divided into two halves, F_1 and F_2, the two subscales serving two purposes. They allow for the identification of infrequent responding when only the first 350 items are administered and only the clinical scales are scored. And they provide a comparison of the adolescent's approach to the first and second halves of the test. Marked (more than 20 T–score points) discrepancies in which F_2 is much greater than F_1 indicate that a substantial change occurred over the course of the test administration and that the quality of data obtained from the second half of the booklet may be compromised. This may be due to a loss of motivation or concentration. Because only the new content and supplementary scales have items in the second half of the booklet, it remains possible, in such cases, to interpret the clinical scales.

Overall, the F scale is designed to identify unusual test protocols. An adolescent who scores higher than 80 on F has provided a very unusual set of responses, and several interpretive possibilities should be considered. The first is random responding. This includes either intentional random responding, in which the adolescent simply marks the answer sheet or presses the keyboard items without pausing to read and respond to the content of the items, or unintentional random responding that may occur when the adolescent cannot read or comprehend the items either because of limited abilities or severe confusion or disorientation.

A second possible reason for elevated scores on F is that the adolescent has very severe behavioral problems, psychopathology, and/or emotional distress. Because such severe problems tend to be relatively rare in adolescents, they are represented by the Infrequency Scale items, in particular those on F_1 that come from the clinical scales. An adolescent who experiences severe behavioral, emotional, or other problems will produce an elevated score on F and often a pattern of scores in which F_1 is greater than F_2.

A third possible reason for elevation on the F scale is an intentional attempt by the test–takers to over–report their problems and to appear worse than they actually are.

Such an approach, termed "Fake Bad," will result in an elevated score on this scale. The primary task of the test interpreter when confronted by an elevated score on F is to determine the extent to which each of these three factors has played a role in a given protocol. The factors are not mutually exclusive and may all be operating to varying degrees in a given case.

If an adolescent who has produced an elevated score on F has an extensive history of serious emotional problems, the role of severe dysfunction in elevating the score on this scale needs to be weighed relatively heavily. Conversely, if an adolescent has no prior history of severe problems, and is doing fairly well living at home and attending school, it becomes less likely that this factor has played a role in elevating this scale score. The role of random responding in an elevated score on the F scale can be discerned from one of the new MMPI–A validity scales, VRIN, discussed below.

The K Scale

Like L, K is one of the original MMPI validity scales. It was developed by Paul Meehl after the original instrument had been completed, in response to recurring cases in which an individual presented with clearly evident symptoms of psychopathology, yet produced a "normal" MMPI profile. It is designed to measure the degree to which a test–taker has taken a defensive approach in responding to the test. In adults, a correction factor, the K–correction, is added to several of the clinical scales to account for the effects of defensiveness.

Because research with adolescents has failed to support the utility of the K–correction with this population, the correction was not incorporated in the MMPI–A. However, the scale itself remains and T scores above 65 are indicative of a defensive approach to the test. An important caveat in interpreting this scale stems from the fact that, like L, all but one of the 30 K items are keyed false. Therefore, the same concerns regarding the effects of response sets on L scores apply to scores on K.

Again, the new validity scale TRIN is of vital importance in identifying the occurrence of nay- or yea-saying.

Variable Response Inconsistency

The Variable Response Inconsistency Scale (VRIN) is an MMPI–A scale designed to identify and quantify random responding. It is made up of item pairs that are either nearly identical or nearly opposite in meaning. It is keyed so that an inconsistent response of any combination (True–True, True–False, False–True, or False–False) might produce a raw score point on this scale. Item pairs were identified initially through statistical analyses and verified subsequently through conceptual analyses to ensure that inconsistency is both statistical and conceptual. T scores greater than 75 on this scale are indicative of an excessive amount of random responding that jeopardizes the integrity of the test protocol.

True Response Inconsistency

The True Response Inconsistency scale (TRIN) is also made up of item pairs and is designed to identify the response sets of yea–saying, indiscriminant true responding, and nay–saying, indiscriminant false responding. It is made up of items that are opposite in meaning so that a pattern of "True" or "False" responses to both items in a pair indicates indiscriminant responding in the direction of the response (true or false).

Scoring of this scale is somewhat complicated. The number of inconsistent "True" and "False" responses is counted separately, and the raw score is calculated to produce a T score that will never be lower than 50. Any T score greater than 50 is followed by either a "T" or an "F," indicating a predominant pattern of inconsistent "True" or "False" responding. A T score greater than 100 on this scale (in either direction) indicates an excessive level of inconsistent responding that likely invalidates the resulting profile.

TRIN is particularly important in evaluating scores on scales such as L and K that are keyed predominantly in one direction (for these two scales, "False"). The effects of yea–saying and nay–saying, although not limited to scales with a predominant scoring direction, are most notable on such scales. Whenever highly deviant (very low or very high) scores are observed on L and K, the score on TRIN should be examined to rule in, or out, the possible effects of a response set.

Clinical Scales

The original MMPI clinical scales remain, for the most part, unchanged insofar as their composition on the MMPI–A is concerned. Scales 3, 6, 7, and 9 are unchanged, with the exception of several items that were rewritten for the MMPI–A (Archer & Gordon, 1994; Williams, Ben–Porath, & Hevren, 1994).[3] Scales 1, 4, and 8 lost one item, Scale 2 lost three items, Scale 0 lost eight items, and Scale 5 lost 16 items. With the exception of the last two scales, items were omitted if they were deemed to contain objectionable content. For scales 0 and 5, items that were scored only on either of these scales and, for scale 5, items that did not differentiate statistically between boys and girls in the normative sample, were deleted from the scale in the interest of reducing the length of the inventory.

Data reported in the MMPI–A manual include up–to–date empirical correlates for the slightly reconstituted clinical scales. These correlates, derived from the normative and clinical samples described previously, are consistent with past findings. Following are brief descriptions of the MMPI–A clinical scales.

Scale 1 — Hypochondriasis (Hs)[4]

Scale 1 is a measure of pre–occupation with health concerns. In addition to somatic concerns, elevated[5] scores on this scale indicate that an adolescent may be having academic problems and has a tendency toward internalizing behaviors, including being fearful, guilt–prone, and withdrawn. Girls may also have eating problems.

Scale 2 — Depression (D)

Elevated scores on this scale are associated with depression, feelings of guilt and pessimism, and the presence of suicidal ideation. Adolescents who score high on this scale tend to lack self–confidence and to be shy and socially withdrawn.

Scale 3 — Hysteria (Hy)

Elevated scores on this scale are associated with somatic concerns, immaturity, self–centeredness, and a need for attention and affection. Adolescents who score high on this scale also tend to lack insight into their problems and behavior.

Scale 4 — Psychopathic Deviate (Pd)

High scores on this scale are associated with various acting-out behaviors, including behavioral problems at school and within the family and conflicts with figures of authority. Substance use and abuse are more likely in adolescents who score high on this scale as are impulsive and aggressive behaviors. Research reported in the MMPI–A manual suggests that adolescent boys in clinical settings who score high on this scale are at greater risk for having been physically abused, whereas adolescent girls who produce elevated scores are at greater risk for having been sexually abused.[6]

Scale 5 — Masculinity–Femininity (Mf)

Boys who score high on this scale are more likely to possess stereotypically feminine and less likely to possess stereotypically masculine interests. They also are less likely to engage in acting-out behaviors. An opposite pattern is expected for girls who score high on this scale. They will more likely have stereotypically masculine interests, they are less likely to have stereotypically feminine interests, and they are more likely to engage in acting-out behaviors.

Scale 6 — Paranoia (Pa)

Elevated scores on this scale are associated with heightened suspiciousness and mistrust, and greater sensitivity to perceived criticism and rejection. Adolescents who score high on this scale tend to blame others for their problems. At extreme levels of elevation, paranoid delusional thinking may be present.

Scale 7 — Psychasthenia (Pt)

High scores on this scale are associated with the presence of anxiety, depression, and emotional turmoil. Adolescents who produce elevations on this scale tend to lack self–confidence and to be highly self–critical. They may also have difficulties making decisions. Research reported in the MMPI–A manual indicates that adolescent boys who score high on this scale are at increased risk for having been sexually abused.

Scale 8 — Schizophrenia (Sc)

Elevated scores on this scale are associated with extreme psychological turmoil, behavioral acting-out tendencies, social and emotional alienation, and hyper–sensitivity to stress. High scorers on this scale are at increased risk for substance use and abuse and they tend to have low self–esteem. Those who produce highly elevated scores on this scale may present with frankly psychotic symptoms.

Scale 9 — Hypomania (Ma)

Elevated scores on this scale are associated with acting-out tendencies, impulsive behavior, and problems with authority. Adolescents who score high on this scale are at increased risk for substance use and abuse. Very high scores may indicate the presence of manic or hypomanic symptoms.

Scale 0 — Social Introversion (Si)

This scale measures the construct of extraversion–introversion. Elevated scores indicate that an adolescent tends to be shy and withdrawn, and likely has difficulties forming friendships. Low scores on this scale (particularly below a T score of 40), indicate that an adolescent tends to be extraverted and very comfortable in social situations.

As indicated at the outset of this section, this brief description of the clinical scales is intended to provide the reader with a general overview of what they measure. Test interpreters who are not very familiar with these scales should consult one of the interpretive guides identified previously. These sources also provide information regarding subscales that are available to assist in the interpretation of the clinical scales. These scales, developed primarily by Harris and Lingoes (1955) for several of the clinical scales, and more recently by Ben–Porath, Hostetler, Butcher, and Graham (1989) for Scale 0, assist in the interpretation of the clinical scales by dividing them into content–homogeneous clusters. A list of these scales is found in Table 1. Their use is illustrated in several of the cases presented in this book.

Content Scales

The MMPI–A Content Scales (Williams, Butcher, Ben–Porath, & Graham, 1992) were developed in the tradition of the Wiggins (1966) content scales for the original MMPI. They were constructed by a series of rational and statistical analyses that were designed to produce reliable, content–based measures of adolescent functioning in a number of areas. Complete details on their development and psychometric properties are provided by Williams et al. (1992). We present here a brief description of the 15 scales.

Adolescent Anxiety (A–anx)

This scale contains items that describe various symptoms of anxiety including tension, frequent worrying, and fears of losing control. Adolescents who score high on this scale are prone to excessive worry and anxiety.

Adolescent Obsessiveness (A–obs)

Adolescents who produce elevated scores on this scale are reporting a large number of obsessive–compulsive tendencies. They tend to ruminate and have significant difficulties making decisions and changes in their lives.

Adolescent Depression (A–dep)

Youngsters who score high on this scale report many symptoms of depression including sadness, crying, self–depreciatory thinking, and fatigue. They may also be reporting suicidal tendencies.

Table 1

Subscales for the MMPI-A Clinical Scales

Harris Lingoes (1955) Subscales

Scale 2
   D$_1$ Subjective Depression
   D$_2$ Psychomotor Retardation
   D$_3$ Physical Malfunctioning
   D$_4$ Mental Dullness
   D$_5$ Brooding

Scale 3
   Hy$_1$ Denial of Social Anxiety
   Hy$_2$ Need for Affection
   Hy$_3$ Lassitude–Malaise
   Hy$_4$ Somatic Complaints
   Hy$_5$ Inhibition of Aggression

Scale 4
   Pd$_1$ Familial Discord
   Pd$_2$ Authority Problems
   Pd$_3$ Social Imperturbability
   Pd$_4$ Social Alienation
   Pd$_5$ Self–Alienation

Scale 6
   Pa$_1$ Persecutory Ideas
   Pa$_2$ Poignancy
   Pa$_3$ Naivete

Scale 8
   Sc$_1$ Social Alienation
   Sc$_2$ Emotional Alienation
   Sc$_3$ Lack of Ego Mastery, Cognitive
   Sc$_4$ Lack of Ego Mastery, Conative
   Sc$_5$ Lack of Ego Mastery, Defective Inhibition
   Sc$_6$ Bizarre Sensory Experiences

Scale 9
   Ma$_1$ Amorality
   Ma$_2$ Psychomotor Acceleration
   Ma$_3$ Imperturbability
   Ma$_4$ Ego Inflation

Scale 0 (Ben–Porath, Hostetler, Butcher, & Graham, 1989)
   Si$_1$ Shyness/Self–consciousness
   Si$_2$ Social Avoidance
   Si$_3$ Self/Other Alienation

Adolescent Health Concerns (A–hea)

Adolescents who score high on this scale report a large number of physical health concerns and they are generally worried about their health.

Adolescent Alienation (A–aln)

Adolescents who produce elevated scores on this scale report experiencing considerable emotional distance from others. They feel that they cannot get close to other people and cannot turn to others for support.

Adolescent Bizarre Mentation (A–biz)

Youngsters who produce elevated scores on this scale report very unusual, generally psychotic symptoms. They may be experiencing delusional thinking and hallucinations.

Adolescent Anger (A–ang)

Elevated scores on this scale indicate that an adolescent has reported problems with anger management and control. A high-scoring adolescent is likely to be irritable and may tend toward explosive outbursts.

Adolescent Cynicism (A–cyn)

High scores on this scale indicate that an adolescent has reported a large number of misanthropic beliefs and is generally guarded and suspicious in interpersonal relationships.

Adolescent Conduct Problems (A–con)

Youngsters who score high on this scale report engaging in a large number of acting-out behaviors, including stealing, lying, and various illegal acts.

Adolescent Low Self–Esteem (A–lse)

High scores on this scale indicate that an adolescent reports having a negative self–view, being interpersonally submissive, and having little confidence in him- or herself.

Adolescent Low Aspirations (A–las)

Elevated scores on this scale indicate that an adolescent has reported having very low expectations for her/his future, not engaging in activities designed to improve her- or himself, and a tendency to give up easily when things go wrong.

Adolescent Social Discomfort (A–sod)

Adolescents who score high on this scale report being very uncomfortable in social situations. They tend to avoid such situations whenever possible.

Adolescent Family Problems (A–fam)

Youngsters who produce elevated scores on this scale indicate that they have significant conflicts within their family, they are dissatisfied with their family life and believe that they cannot count on their family for help and support.

Adolescent School Problems (A–sch)

Elevated scores on this scale indicate that an adolescent has reported having a large number of disciplinary and academic problems in school.

Adolescent Negative Treatment Indicators (A–trt)

High scores on this scale indicate that a youngster has reported holding various views, attitudes, and beliefs that may interfere with his or her treatment. These may include low motivation for treatment, distrust of health professionals, and general pessimism regarding their potential to succeed in therapy.

Supplementary Scales

Six additional measures, termed "supplementary," are included among the MMPI–A scales that are normed and reported in the test manual. Some were newly developed for the MMPI–A, others are adaptations of original MMPI scales.

MacAndrew Alcoholism Scale — Revised (MAC–R)

This original MMPI scale has been modified slightly for the MMPI–A. It measures personality factors that place an adolescent at increased risk for developing a substance-use problem. It is associated with tendencies toward sensation–seeking and impulsivity.

Alcohol/Drug Problem Proneness Scale (PRO)

This is a newly developed (Weed et al.

1994) MMPI–A scale that, like MAC–R, measures personality traits that place an adolescent at increased risk for developing a substance-use problem. PRO differs from MAC–R in that it incorporates many items that were newly written for the MMPI–A and it appears to be associated more strongly with a susceptibility to negative peer-group influences.

Alcohol/Drug Problem Acknowledgment Scale (ACK)

This is also a newly developed (Weed et al., 1994) MMPI–A scale designed to assess substance-use problems. Unlike MAC–R and PRO, it is made up of items that deal directly with the acknowledgment of substance-use problems. Research indicates that it is the strongest predictor of problematic use patterns among the three substance-use scales.

Immaturity (IMM)

This is a newly developed (Archer, Pancoast, & Gordon, 1994) MMPI–A scale designed to assess psychological maturation during adolescence using Loevinger's concept of ego development.

Anxiety (A)

This is a slightly modified version of the original MMPI Welsh (1956) Anxiety scale. Elevated scores indicate the presence of anxiety, depression, pessimism, and perfectionism.

Repression (R)

This is a slightly modified version of the original MMPI Welsh (1956) Repression scale. It is associated with emotional over–control.

Notes

1. The lower boundary of age 14 is recommended in the MMPI–A manual (Butcher et al., 1992) based on data analyses conducted in the development of the instrument that suggested a qualitative drop in the validity of test data provided by adolescents 13 years old and younger. However, because the data analyzed were collected with an experimental, 704–item version of the instrument, it is possible that 13-year-olds may be capable of providing more valid information when completing the 478–item final version of the MMPI–A. Archer (1992) provides MMPI–A norms for 13-year-olds based on a limited set of data. We recommend that clinicians who administer the MMPI–A not score the profiles of 13-year-olds with these norms. Rather, we recommend that they be scored on the complete set of norms provided in the test manual, and that the validity scales, particularly VRIN (see next section), be examined carefully to determine whether the data are interpretable. If they are, test interpretation can proceed with caution.

2. Throughout this section we identify cutoffs for the determination of profile validity. However, we urge the reader to view these recommended cutoffs as general interpretive guidelines. In the case of Cannot Say, for example, 29 item omissions are generally as problematic as 31, and both are far less problematic than, say, 50. In general, the higher the score on a validity indicator, the greater the likelihood that the protocol is uninterpretable.

3. Archer and Gordon (1994) and Williams et al. (1994) conducted studies of the effects of rewriting MMPI–A items on the psychometric functioning of the scales. Items on the MMPI–A were rewritten to correct awkward and gender-specific language and to change content describing adolescents' experiences from the past to the present tense. The goal was to improve the readability and face validity of the instrument without affecting the actual functioning of the scales. These authors

found, as expected, that improvements in language did not alter the psychometric functioning of the scales on which they were scored.

4. Throughout this book, we refer (following Graham, 1993) to the clinical scales primarily by their numeric designator. The original scale names and abbreviations are noted here for identification purposes only. It is our view that it is preferable to use the numeric designator so as not to confuse the original scale labels with the constructs that are actually measured by these scales.

5. In general, T scores greater than 60 are considered elevated on the MMPI-A clinical, content, and supplementary scales. The same caveat regarding over-reliance on cutoff scores raised in reference to the validity scales applies to these scales and this cutoff as well.

6. Greater risk for abuse should not be interpreted as an indication or confirmation that abuse has actually occurred. It suggests the need for follow-up in this area.

References

Achenbach, T. M., & Edlebrock, C. S. (1983). *Manual for the Child Behavior Checklist and Revised Child Profile.* Burlington, VT: University of Vermont, Department of Psychiatry.

Archer, R. P. (1987). *Using the MMPI with adolescents.* Hillsdale, NJ: Lawrence Erlbaum & Associates.

Archer, R. P. (1992). *MMPI-A: Assessing adolescent psychopathology.* Hillsdale, NJ: Lawrence Erlbaum & Associates.

Archer, R. P., & Gordon, R. (1994). Psychometric stability of MMPI-A item modifications. *Journal of Personality Assessment, 62,* 416-426.

Archer, R. P., Pancoast, D. L., & Gordon, R. A. (1994). The development of the MMPI-A Immaturity Scale: Findings from normal and clinical samples. *Journal of Personality Assessment, 62,* 145-156.

Ben-Porath, Y. S., Hostetler, K., Butcher, J. N., & Graham, J. R. (1989). New subscales for the MMPI Social Introversion (Si) scale. *Psychological Assessment, 1,* 169-174.

Ben-Porath, Y. S., Williams, C. L., & Uchiyama, C. (1989). New scales for the Devereux Adolescent Behavior Rating scale. *Psychological Assessment, 1,* 58-60.

Butcher, J. N., Dahlstrom, W. G., Graham, J. R., Tellegen, A., & Kaemmer, B. (1989). *Minnesota Multiphasic Personality Inventory-2: Manual for administration and scoring.* Minneapolis, MN: University of Minnesota Press.

Butcher, J. N., Graham, J. R., Williams, C. L., Archer, R. P., Tellegen, A., Ben-Porath, Y. S., & Kaemmer, B. (1992). *Minnesota Multiphasic Personality Inventory - Adolescent: Manual for scoring and interpretation.* Minneapolis, MN: University of Minnesota Press.

Butcher, J. N., & Williams, C. L. (1992). *Essentials of MMPI-2 and MMPI-A interpretation.* Minneapolis, MN: University of Minnesota Press.

Capwell, D. F. (1945a). Personality patterns of adolescent girls I. Girls who show no improvement in IQ. *Journal of Applied Psychology, 29,* 212-228.

Capwell, D. F. (1945b). Personality patterns of adolescent girls II. Delinquents and nondelinquents. *Journal of Applied Psychology, 29,* 289-297.

Dahlstrom, W. G., Welsh, G. S., & Dahlstrom, L. E. (1972). *An MMPI handbook: Volume I, Clinical interpretation.* Minneapolis, MN: University of Minnesota Press.

Graham, J. R. (1993). MMPI-2: *Assessing personality and psychopathology, second edition.* New York, NY: Oxford University Press.

Harris, R. E., & Lingoes, J. C. (1955). *Subscales for the MMPI: An aid to interpretation.* Unpublished document.

Hathaway, S. R., & McKinley, J. C. (1943). *Minnesota Multiphasic Personality*

Inventory. Minneapolis, MN: University of Minnesota Press.

Hathaway, S. R., & Monachesi, E. D. (1953). *Analyzing and predicting juvenile delinquency with the MMPI*. Minneapolis, MN: University of Minnesota Press.

Hathaway, S. R., & Monachesi, E. D. (1957). The personalities of pre–delinquent boys. *Journal of Criminal Law, Criminology, and Political Science, 48,* 149–153.

Hathaway, S. R., & Monachesi, E. D. (1963). *Adolescent personality and Behavior: MMPI patterns of normal, delinquent, drop–out, and other outcomes*. Minneapolis, MN: University of Minnesota Press.

Marks, P. A., Seeman, W., & Haller, D. L. (1974). *The actuarial use of the MMPI with adolescents*. Baltimore, MD: Williams and Wilkins.

Meehl, P. E. (1954). *Clinical versus statistical prediction: A theoretical analysis and a review of the evidence*. Minneapolis, MN: University of Minnesota Press.

Weed, N. C., Butcher, J. N., & Williams, C. L. (1994). Development of an MMPI–A alcohol/drug problem scale. *Journal of Studies on Alcohol, 55,* 296–302.

Welsh, G. S. (1956). Factor dimensions A and R. In G. S. Welsh & W. G. Dahlstrom (Eds.), *Basic readings on the MMPI in psychology and medicine*. Minneapolis, MN: University of Minnesota Press.

Wiggins, J. S. (1966). Substantive dimensions of self-report in the MMPI item pool. *Psychological Monographs, 80* (22, Whole No. 630).

Williams, C. L., Ben–Porath, Y. S., & Hevren, V. W. (1994). Item level improvements for use of the MMPI with adolescents. *Journal of Personality Assessment, 63,* 284–293.

Williams, C. L., & Butcher, J. N. (1989). An MMPI study of adolescents: I. Empirical validity of the standard scales. *Psychological Assessment, 1,* 251–259.

Williams, C. L., Butcher, J. N., Ben–Porath, Y. S., & Graham, J. R. (1992). *MMPI–A Content Scales: Assessing psychopathology in adolescents*. Minneapolis, MN: University of Minnesota Press.

AN INTERPRETIVE STRATEGY FOR THE MMPI–A

In this chapter, we present the strategy for MMPI–A interpretation that we followed in this book. The approach we use and recommend is fashioned after the strategy described by Graham (1993) for interpreting MMPI–2 and MMPI–A profiles. An MMPI–A interpretation based on this approach addresses five areas:

- Profile validity
- Current level of adjustment
- Symptoms and traits
- Diagnostic suggestions
- Treatment recommendations

In the following sections we discuss what should be included in each area of interpretation and the sources for this information. Once more, our emphasis on interpreting profile validity reflects our view that this is the single most important aspect of MMPI–A interpretation.

PROFILE VALIDITY

The first part of any MMPI–A interpretation should provide the reader with information regarding the validity of the individual test profile. Although it may seem unnecessary to address this in a clinical casebook, it is important to emphasize the difference between profile validity and test validity. *Test validity* is a psychometric concept that refers to the ability of a psychometric scale to measure what it is intended to measure. It typically is established through studies involving large numbers of individuals.

Profile validity, on the other hand, refers to the quality of information contained in a specific set of scores produced by an individual. A test could hypothetically be 100% valid, yet if the person taking it responds randomly, the resulting scores are 100% useless, or invalid. Thus, for any given test administration, the validity of the data generated by the individual taking the test needs to be weighed and considered.

It is, in our view, a mistake to view and treat profile validity as a dichotomous variable whereby a test is either valid or invalid. A more sophisticated view treats profile validity as a continuous dimension, ranging from valid to invalid, with quantifiable gradations between the two extremes of the dimension. Moreover, with respect to self–report instruments, there are several different potential threats to profile validity, each of which may be considered along a continuous scale.

Two broad classes of threats to profile validity are random and non–random responding. *Random responding* occurs when the test–taker answers the test items indiscriminantly and nonsystematically, without considering and understanding them. It includes, but is not limited to, cases where an individual intentionally fails to read the test items and indicates her or his responses randomly. Random responding also occurs when the test–taker attempts but is unable to understand the test items and nevertheless responds to them. This may happen in situations where the adolescent has reading and/or comprehension problems, or if he or she is confused or disorganized.

AN INTERPRETIVE STRATEGY

As described in the introduction, the validity scale VRIN measures the extent to which random responding has occurred in a given profile. And, as also discussed in the introduction, although a T score of 75 is recommended as the cutoff for excessive random responding that likely invalidates the resulting profile, a T score of 74 on this scale is essentially equally problematic. Sophisticated interpretation of scores on this as well as the other validity scales takes into account various levels of invalidity. Thus, in a case where an adolescent produces a T score of 70 on VRIN, it is possible to interpret the resulting test scores. However, considerable caution must be exercised not to over–interpret any particularly abnormal patterns or scores.

Non–random invalid responding occurs when the test-taker somehow distorts his or her responses in a systematic way. There are, essentially, two types of systematic invalid responding. The first is *Fixed Responding*, which involves the response sets identified earlier as yea-saying and nay-saying. Here, the test–taker responds to the items in a fixed, rather than random, manner. However, the responses are not based on the content of the test items. Rather, they involve a pattern of indiscriminant "True" or "False" responding. As described in the introduction, the MMPI–A TRIN scale identifies and quantifies fixed responding when it occurs. Like random responding, fixed responding may occur to varying degrees and with different effects in a given profile.

The second type of non–random, invalid responding is *Misleading Responding*. Here, responses are based on the content of test items. However, the test-taker responds in a manner that is designed (usually, but not always, intentionally) to mislead the test interpreter. Misleading responding, by definition, cannot be random or inconsistent because it requires that the test–taker read, understand, and respond (in a misleading manner) to the test items. Thus, highly elevated scores on either VRIN or TRIN rule out the possibility of misleading responding.

Two general types of misleading responding have been described in the literature as *Fake Bad* and *Fake Good*. Fake Bad involves a pattern of responding in which individuals describe themselves as having more severe problems than they actually have. In extreme cases, the adolescent may fabricate problems that do not exist. In less severe cases, he or she may exaggerate the severity of problems that do exist. The F scales are good measures of the Fake Bad approach.

Fake Good is a pattern of responding characterized by denying or minimizing problems. Denial refers to situations in which test–takers fail to report problems they are experiencing, whereas minimization involves acknowledging problems, yet downplaying their severity or impact. Highly elevated scores on the L scale have traditionally been associated with denial, whereas elevations on K are typically associated with minimization.

In describing profile validity, then, the test–interpreter conducts a systematic appraisal of scores on the validity scales. When these scales are elevated, the meaning of a particular pattern of invalid responding is considered and conclusions are drawn regarding the impact of such responding on scores on the remaining scales. In extreme cases, a profile may be determined to be completely invalid or uninterpretable. In less severe cases, concerns may be raised and interpretation may proceed with caution.

Finally, information concerning profile validity may be gleaned from sources beyond the validity scales. Behavioral observations may sometimes be very informative. For example, if an adolescent completes an MMPI–A in, say, under 20 minutes, there is a very strong likelihood that he or she has not responded very carefully to the test items. On the other hand, if an adolescent takes an unusually long time (over two hours) to complete the test, and in the course of testing frequently asks for assistance in reading and understanding the test items, there is a substantial likelihood that random responding owing to reading and comprehension problems may have occurred.

It is noteworthy that both situations just described will result in elevated scores on VRIN, and it is only by reliance on behavioral observations that the test–interpreter may gain an understanding that random responding resulted in an invalid profile. This underscores the importance of monitoring the administration of the MMPI–A. It is, in our view, an unacceptable practice to have adolescents (or adults) complete the MMPI–A without supervision.

We have not included any completely invalid cases in this book. However, several of the cases illustrate how a test–interpreter deals with situations where a profile is less than 100% valid, yet can still be used to generate useful interpretive information.

GENERAL LEVEL OF ADJUSTMENT

The next area to be covered in an MMPI–A interpretation is the adolescent's general level of adjustment. Here, global statements are made about the youngster's overall functioning. This can range from an adolescent who appears to be better adjusted than average to one who is experiencing severe psychological turmoil and is likely to be incapable of caring for her- or himself. The adolescent's level or degree of emotional distress, as well as whether and how this distress is affecting his or her ability to fulfill major role obligations will be the focus of interpretation.

The MMPI–A provides several sources of information regarding an adolescent's general level of adjustment. Assuming that a profile has been found to be valid, the score on F is one of the more sensitive MMPI–A indicators of general adjustment or maladjustment. The higher the score on F, the more likely it is that the adolescent is having substantial, or, at higher levels of elevation, severe problems. These may involve the experience of psychotic symptoms.

On the clinical profile, scales 2 and 7 tend to be the most "state–dependent" in that they vary the most as a function of an

adolescent's current level of distress. Scale 8 is also sensitive to distress. However, it is, in addition, related to more chronic problems and is therefore a less sensitive indicator of current dysfunction. The sensitivity to distress of scales 2 and 7 also means that as an adolescent's condition improves, these are the scale scores that are most likely to change, and thus reflect improvement.

Another indicator of general level of adjustment is the adolescent's mean score on the clinical scales. Typically this number is provided by computerized scoring services. A related, more crude indicator of general functioning is the number of clinical scales that are elevated above the threshold for clinically meaningful elevation, a T score of 60. Similar conclusions may be drawn from the mean score and number of elevated scales on the MMPI–A Content Scales profile.

A final clinical scale indicator of general level of adjustment is the *slope* of the MMPI–A profile. This refers to whether the pattern of scores across the profile is such that they tend either to increase or decrease systematically.

A positive slope is one in which most of the clinically significant elevation occurs in the latter part of the profile, particularly on scales 6, 8, and 9. This pattern indicates very substantial psychological distress and the likelihood that the adolescent feels overwhelmed and unable to cope with his or her difficulties. A negative slope occurs when the highest elevations are found on the left–hand side of the profile, particularly on scales 1, 2, and 3, sometimes called the "neurotic triad." This pattern suggests less severe, but more chronic maladjustment. Examples of both types of slope are found among the cases in this book.

Finally, the supplementary Welsh Anxiety Scale, A, is also one of the more sensitive MMPI–A indicators of general maladjustment. Overall, the greater the number of these indicators that point toward a given conclusion (e.g., severe turmoil and distress), the greater the confidence that can be placed in the interpretation.

SYMPTOMS AND TRAITS

In this part of the interpretation, information is gleaned from the entire set of MMPI–A scales to indicate which, if any, symptoms of psychopathology are likely present and which personality traits and behavioral tendencies are indicated. Specific issues that may be addressed include:

■ The presence of symptoms of depression, anxiety, psychosis, or conduct problems.

■ The manner in which the adolescent tends to perceive his or her environment (e.g., supportive versus threatening).

■ Whether this youngster is inclined to over–react to stressful situations.

■ The nature of the adolescent's self–concept.

■ Whether this youngster is emotionally over– or under–controlled.

■ How this young person relates interpersonally.

All of the MMPI–A scales serve as potential sources of information for this section. However, more often than not the test will not yield information to address each of these issues. In general, interpretation should proceed from the clinical scales, to the content scales, and, finally, to the supplementary scales. Conflicts, if they arise, should be resolved by relying on the indicator that has greater established empirical validity and with appropriate qualification of the particular interpretive statement. Redundancy, that is similar interpretations suggested by different scales, should lead to greater confidence in a particular interpretation.

Often, the section on symptoms and traits will be the richest and longest component of the MMPI–A report. The interpretive references cited in the introduction may serve as the primary source for deriving empirically based statements for this section.

DIAGNOSTIC SUGGESTIONS

In this part of the report, the test–interpreter proposes for further consideration possible diagnoses that are suggested by the test scores. Although the MMPI was developed initially to point directly toward specific psychiatric diagnoses, users of the test have long recognized that, like all other self–report measures, the MMPI falls short of being able to predict diagnoses with sufficient accuracy to generate them directly from test scores.

This "shortcoming" of self–report measures, in our view, is attributable more to the unreliable nature of psychiatric diagnosis than to inherent difficulties of assessment by self–report. Regardless of its cause, the weak predictive power of MMPI (and MMPI–A) scales in reference to specific psychiatric diagnoses argues against using the test to derive specific diagnoses. Nevertheless, diagnostic suggestions can and should be offered on the basis of MMPI–A scale scores.

Diagnostic suggestions identify psychiatric diagnoses that *may* be present, but require additional exploration and interviewing to confirm. They may be based either on data that indicate a correlation between an MMPI–A score and a certain diagnosis or on inferences based on the suggestion that certain symptoms and behaviors are present.

An example of the former are clinical Scale 2 and content scale Adolescent Depression (A–dep), both of which are correlated significantly with depression. Thus, if one (and even more so if both) of these scales is elevated, the interpreter can raise the possibility of a depressive disorder being present. The greater the elevation, the greater the likelihood that such a condition does, in fact, exist. An example of the latter is a profile that indicates the presence of emotional lability, suicidal ideation, anger management problems, and poor self– esteem, which may, by inference, be interpreted to *suggest* the presence of a borderline personality disorder. In both cases, the diagnostic suggestions will be presented as such and recommended for follow–up examination.

Sources of information for this section of the interpretation include, once more, all of the clinical, content, and supplementary scales. On a broad level, positive and negative slopes (see above under general level of adjustment) on the clinical scale profile suggest different types of diagnoses. A positive slope is suggestive of a possible psychotic disorder whereas a negative slope indicates the greater likelihood of a neurotic disorder.

Particular attention should be paid in this section to the MMPI–A substance-use scales discussed earlier. For example, an elevated score on the MacAndrew Alcoholism Scale–Revised (MAC–R) (generally any raw score greater than 28 for adolescent boys and 26 for girls) is interpreted to indicate that an adolescent is at *increased risk* for the development of problems in this area. The interpretation of elevated scores on this scale should focus on tendencies toward thrill- and sensation–seeking, which, in turn, increase the risk for problems with substance use. An elevated score (above T score 60) on the Alcohol/Drug Proneness (PRO) scale also indicates a greater risk for problematic substance use. In this instance, however, data suggest that the instigator more likely may be another teen who uses these substances (i.e., negative peer-group influences), rather than any internal pressures.

In both instances, it is, once more, inappropriate to draw any direct diagnostic inferences regarding substance abuse on the basis of MMPI–A scores alone. Research indicates that although correlated with substance-use problems, these scales are not sufficiently powerful to generate specific diagnostic predictions. Thus, it is more appropriate to interpret these scales as indicating the degree of risk for substance abuse.

TREATMENT RECOMMENDATIONS

The final section of an MMPI–A interpretive report will typically (although not always) include treatment recommendations. These may focus on areas of functioning in particular need of attention and intervention, suggested treatment modalities, and the prognosis for a successful outcome.

Areas in need of treatment will typically have already been identified in the sections on symptoms and traits and diagnostic suggestions. Here, the task of the interpreter is to integrate this information and identify for the reader a list of potential treatment targets or goals. Priorities for treatment may also be suggested.

Recommended treatment modalities will depend upon the types of problems identified and the adolescent's personality characteristics. For youngsters experiencing psychotic or major depressive symptoms, a psychiatric evaluation to determine the need for medication may be suggested. For adolescents who appear on the basis of their MMPI–A scores to have little capacity for insight and introspection, insight–oriented therapy may be counter–indicated. For teens with severe anger and behavior-control problems, contingency–based behavioral interventions may be recommended.

Finally, some statements regarding the likely outcome of intervention may be provided. Research has indicated that individuals who, based on their MMPI profile, appear to be experiencing substantial psychological distress are more motivated than others to engage in therapy and are therefore more likely to reap its benefits. Conversely, adolescents who produce profiles suggestive of anti–social tendencies are far less likely to benefit from treatment though they may engage in therapy initially because of an outside incentive or threat.

As can be gleaned from our discussion of treatment recommendations, information for this section may come from any scale on the MMPI–A profile. Validity scale scores indicating defensiveness, clinical scale scores indicating substantial distress, or content scale scores indicating extreme acting-out tendencies may all suggest a specific set of recommendations and prognostications.

One measure, the MMPI–A content scale Adolescent Negative Treatment Indicators (A–trt), was designed specifically to address treatment issues. However, it is sometimes mistaken as a prognostic scale designed to predict treatment outcome. The A–trt scale was not designed for this purpose, and research with the adult version of this scale indicates that it indeed does not predict outcome successfully.

The A–trt scale was designed to identify individuals who may encounter difficulties in treatment and alert the therapist to the possibility of such problems. Its items deal with issues such as motivation for treatment, ability to self–disclose, feelings toward health–care delivery professionals, and ability to form interpersonal relationships. Thus, an elevated score on this scale is most appropriately interpreted as indicating that a teen may have concerns about therapy or may have certain preconceived notions or resistances that may interfere with treatment. It is best viewed as a risk indicator suggestive of the need for extra care and attention to make certain that the youngster is becoming engaged properly in the therapeutic process.

CONCLUSION

In this chapter, we outlined and described our approach to MMPI–A profile interpretation. As has been stressed previously, successful application of this strategy will require, at least initially, that the interpreter make extensive use of available guides and reference sources for MMPI–A interpretation. Citations for these resources were provided in the introduction. The 16 cases included in this book illustrate many of the interpretive strategies and issues just outlined.

PART

2

MMPI-A
CASES

THE CASES

Following are the 16 cases that are the focus of this book. Cases were selected to represent a broad range of adolescent clients who were evaluated in different types of treatment settings. Included among our cases are adolescents who received inpatient, residential, outpatient, and day-treatment services. For purposes of confidentiality, the names of the youth in these clinical examples and any identifying information have been changed.

The 16 case descriptions follow a standard format. General background information is presented first. This includes the reason for referral, basic demographic characteristics, and as much historical information as was available that could be provided without risk of identifying the youngster. The MMPI–A interpretation follows, and each case description is concluded with outcome information when this was available.

The MMPI–A interpretations provided for each case are, essentially, annotated illustrations of how to go about building an MMPI–A–based report. In them, we provide considerable detail regarding how we derived our interpretive statements. A typical MMPI–A report will not include all of this information. However, our intention here is to demonstrate the process, not simply the product, of profile interpretation.

CASE 1
"ANTHONY"

A QUESTION OF READINESS
FOR A LESS RESTRICTIVE ENVIRONMENT

BACKGROUND

Anthony is a 17–year–old, African–American male who had been living with his mother until his arrest for the murder of his 15–year–old half–sister. Following arrest, he was placed in a detention home and then in a psychiatric hospital.

Anthony was born after a normal pregnancy and birth to a 16–year–old mother. His mother later completed two years of college and entered a successful career in public service. He was raised with an aunt almost as a sibling. He was physically healthy but was temperamentally described as a "difficult child." By contrast, his aunt was described as a pleasant, articulate, and bright girl. Anthony slept poorly and cried frequently at night. Gross motor development was normal, but he was seen at a rehabilitation center for "slow speech" beginning at age two and one-half.

At age three, Anthony was treated with Ritalin for hyperactivity. He was described as evidencing numerous conduct problems and was described as "antisocial." At age five, he transitioned from the rehabilitation center to kindergarten, where he was seen as a responsible child who completed his work and was not considered a behavioral problem.

When he was in the seventh grade, Anthony and his mother moved to their present home which was in a new school district. Shortly after the move, he began to isolate himself from his peers. He attended school but had no friends or social interests. Anthony would return home to watch television, listen to rap music or play with wrestling figures. As he progressed through school, he became increasingly isolated. His grandmother began to worry about his unusual behavior, and shortly after that, he began to act out angrily toward his mother, deliberately breaking her belongings, stealing things and creating a mess in her home. He became sullen, rude toward his mother, and frequently would attempt to ignore her.

In the summer before the homicide, Anthony spent most of his time watching television. Of particular concern to his grandmother was a videotape he made of numerous unrelated television programs that he would watch for hours on end. At home, he became extremely territorial. The family room and television became his room and no one was welcomed into his bedroom. He did not allow anyone to change channels on the television or direct any actions in "his world." Over time, the family accommodated to him and did not challenge this behavior.

The day before the murder, Anthony's 15-year-old half-sister moved into his house so that she could attend a different high school. This move was not discussed with him and was a surprise to Anthony. The half-sister, as well, put her things in his room because she did not yet have a place for them. On the day of the murder, it is reported that she turned on "his TV," changed channels without his permission, picked up the portable telephone without his permission, and began to call friends. She, as well, spoke about the activities she planned to join in school, made derogatory remarks about his grades, and, lastly, laid on his blanket in the family room.

Official police reports indicate that the victim was talking on the telephone with her boyfriend for about an hour. During that hour, she had several brief conversations with Anthony. The boyfriend heard her drop the telephone, scream "Call my house," and then heard several gunshots. The boyfriend called the mother and told her what had happened. She went home and found the victim suffering from several gunshot wounds. Both Anthony and her handgun, a .38 revolver, were missing.

In a forensic interview, Anthony related that he was extremely upset that his half-sister was moving in with him and would attend the same school. He recalled that she had brought a "bag of her stuff to my room." She then turned on the TV and started talking to her boyfriend. He stated that he felt she was going to "take over." He felt scared and nervous and that "my presence wasn't there." He then remembers seeing her pick up his report card and laughing at it. He felt more nervous and scared. He then went and got the gun. He stated that he felt as if he was someone else at the time and that the gun was not real.

Police reports indicate that the victim had suffered numerous gunshot wounds. Anthony ran from the house, reported that he thought about jumping in front of a train but eventually turned himself into the police.

In the forensic psychological evaluation, Anthony was found to evidence a severe degree of psychopathology on the Rorschach. He was described as presenting a productive and vivid protocol. Both form and content were distorted, convolutional, and reflective of delusional thought. Content indicated a perception of interpersonal relationships as threatening and hostile. Responses were marked by confabulation and distortion. Emotional control was seen as quite poor and developmentally delayed. He was seen as extremely emotionally detached. The summary impression of the protocol was a similarity to schizophrenic records, that he had little emotional control in reference to thoughts and feelings, with distorted and delusional thinking. The TAT record was striking in its brevity. Of note was that even Anthony's limited responses were nearly completely unrelated to the events portrayed on the cards. Analysis of the offense found that the shooting was a result of his delusional fear of his half-sister's entering his "domain." Although she had no idea of the threat she posed, her behavior pushed him far past his limited defense mechanisms. Her actions of changing his television channels, going into his room, commenting on his grades, and using the telephone are seemingly "normal and expected" behaviors. However, because of Anthony's thought disorder and delusional system, he became threatened, lost track of the reality of the situation, depersonalized and saw no other way out of the situation but to remove the threat by killing her.

Upon admission to a closed residential treatment center, Anthony was initially seen as withdrawn, noncommunicative, and hostile. The diagnosis was Schizophrenia, Paranoid Type, Subchronic and Conduct Disorder. Anthony was placed on an antipsychotic medication and seen in individual and family therapy. A behavioral program limiting his isolation was implemented. After 18 months, he was viewed as being ready for transfer to an open residential setting. Before transfer to the open residential setting, Anthony completed the MMPI-A.

MMPI–A INTERPRETATION
Profile Validity

Examination of Anthony's validity scale scores (page 34) indicates that he produced a valid MMPI–A profile. He responded to all of the test items and appears to have done so in an honest and open manner. His responses were consistent and he did not show any indications of a true or false response set. Anthony's score on F indicates that he acknowledged having a number of emotional and behavioral problems. The discrepancy between F_1 and F_2 is not great enough to indicate a substantial deviation in his approach to the test between the first and second halves of the booklet. His scores do not suggest that Anthony distorted his self–presentation in a negative or positive manner. Overall, Anthony's validity scale profile indicates that he cooperated with the testing and that the resulting scores on the MMPI–A clinical, content, and supplementary scales will likely yield an accurate appraisal of his current functioning.

Current Level of Adjustment

Anthony's MMPI–A profile indicates that he is experiencing some psychological problems at this time. However, these tend to be rather restricted in nature and they are not causing him to feel overwhelmed or unable to cope with his difficulties. His profile is not characterized by a considerable amount of elevation. On the clinical scales, he produced only one elevation that reached a T score of 60. However, on the content scales he has clinically significant elevation on four scales. His elevation on F indicates that Anthony is likely experiencing some distress at this time. However, he is not likely to report feeling debilitated by his difficulties.

Symptoms and Traits

Anthony produced elevation on only one MMPI–A clinical scale, Scale 1. His moderate level of elevation on this scale indicates that Anthony may be somewhat preoccupied with physical health concerns and bodily functions. In addition to indicat-

ing the possibility of preoccupation with physical health, moderate levels of elevation on this scale also indicate a number of personological and behavioral correlates. Anthony may report experiencing some fatigue or lack of energy and is likely to have a history of poor academic performance in school. Adolescents who produce this pattern of scores on the clinical scales tend to be insecure, fear failure, and they tend to be self–punitive, blaming themselves for their problems. They also tend to be self–centered, demanding, and attention–seeking. Finally, Anthony's elevation on this scale suggests that he tends to be somewhat isolated from other people. Scale 1 does not have any subscales, so it is not possible to refine the interpretation of Anthony's elevation on this scale any further. Because no other clinical scale was elevated, it is inappropriate to interpret his scores on any of the Harris and Lingoes subscales.

Anthony produced several clinically elevated scores on the MMPI–A content scales. His most prominent elevation is on the content scale Adolescent Social Discomfort (A–sod). This score indicates that Anthony reports feeling very uncomfortable around others and that he tends to prefer to be by himself. Anthony likely avoids situations where he might encounter large groups of people, and he becomes distressed when he finds himself in such situations.

Anthony's elevation on Adolescent Bizarre Mentation (A–biz) indicates that he reports experiencing a number of very strange thoughts and experiences that may include delusions and hallucinations. His relatively moderate level of elevation on this scale indicates that Anthony is not necessarily experiencing overwhelming psychotic symptoms at this time. Rather, it is possible that some, or perhaps even most, of his elevation on this scale may be attributable to past experiences since a number of items on A–biz are worded in the past tense. This interpretation is also indicated by the absence of any significant elevation on clinical scales 6 or 8 at this time. However, Anthony's elevation on A–biz does indicate that he is susceptible to psychotic symptomatology.

Anthony's elevation on Adolescent Depression (A–dep) indicates that he reports experiencing some depressive symptomatology at this time. He may report feeling sad and depressed and, as in any case where the MMPI–A indicates depressive symptoms, he may be experiencing suicidal ideation. Examination of the List of Suggested Items for Follow–up (page 38) indicates that Anthony did indeed endorse one suicidal ideation item. This will clearly require immediate follow–up.

Anthony's elevation on the Adolescent School Problems (A–sch) indicates that he reports numerous difficulties in school. Because his level of elevation on this scale is moderate, it is possible that these problems tend to be focussed in one area (e.g., disciplinary or academic).

Anthony's MMPI–A content scale profile contains a number of positive indications. His overall level of elevation on these scales is not indicative of severe problems. Further, his average score on Adolescent Alienation (A–aln) indicates that Anthony is not feeling disengaged from his environment and his average score on Adolescent Negative Treatment Indicators (A–trt) suggests that, in spite of his social uneasiness, Anthony may be open to forming and benefitting from therapeutic relationships. Anthony's within-normal-limits score on Adolescent Low Aspirations (A–las) suggests that he has not given up on himself or his future. Finally, Anthony's average score on Adolescent Health Concerns (A–hea), a more direct measure of an adolescent's preoccupation with physical symptoms than is clinical Scale 1, indicates that the personological correlates of Scale 1 are the most appropriate interpretation of Anthony's elevation on that scale.

Anthony produced an elevated score on one of the MMPI–A supplementary scales, Immaturity. This elevation suggests that Anthony may be emotionally immature for his age and that he may be easily frustrated.

Diagnostic Suggestions

In rendering MMPI–A–based diagnostic suggestions, it is useful to consider the background of the referral. In this case, it is well established that Anthony has had a diagnosed paranoid schizophrenic disorder in the past. His current profile indicates that Anthony's schizophrenic condition is either in remission or, at the very least, is under good control with the aid of medication and psychotherapy. Insofar as the positive symptoms of schizophrenia are concerned, Anthony is not reporting a large number of frankly psychotic symptoms at this time. However, Anthony continues to manifest some of the negative symptoms of this condition, most notably pronounced social discomfort and anhedonia. Anthony's level of social discomfort may, in addition, be reflective of a schizoid personality disorder. Coupled with his moderate elevation on A–biz, Anthony's social discomfort may also be indicative of a schizotypal personality disorder. Although the MMPI–A does not provide sufficient information for differentiation between these diagnostic possibilities, it does suggest the likelihood of a schizophrenia–spectrum disorder.

Anthony's MMPI–A profile also indicates that he continues to report some behavioral acting out and that this pattern may be most prominent at school. Although this indicates the possibility of a conduct disorder, careful consideration needs to be given to whether these behaviors may, to some extent, be explained by Anthony's possible schizophrenia–spectrum disorder.

Finally, Anthony's profile also indicates that he is experiencing some depressed mood and suicidal ideation at this time. Like his acting out, Anthony's mood symptoms may also be related to a possible schizophrenia–spectrum disorder. However, the possibility of a mood disorder or an adjustment disorder with mixed disturbance of emotions and conduct should also be considered.

Treatment Recommendations

Anthony's MMPI–A profile indicates that he continues to be in need of intervention. The nature and severity of his suicidal ideation need to be investigated immediately. Further efforts at controlling his psychotic symptoms with medication and therapy are clearly indicated. As Anthony prepares to leave the locked, intensive-care unit of the facility and to enter the open residential unit, particular attention should be paid to his significant social discomfort. In addition, behavioral modification may be indicated to help Anthony control his outbursts.

OUTCOME

Anthony was transferred to an open, residential unit. He was involved in individual therapy, social-skills training, anger-management groups, life-skills and art therapy. He was placed in the vocational program and prospered in that program. At one point, he discontinued his medication but asked on his own accord to return to it. After one year of continued treatment in the open campus, a series of home visits was begun. Eventually, Anthony returned to his home where he continued to receive individual therapy, family therapy, and anti–psychotic medication.

CASE 1
"ANTHONY"

MMPI-A*

Extended Score Report

ID Number 1

Anthony

Male

Age 17

1/28/93

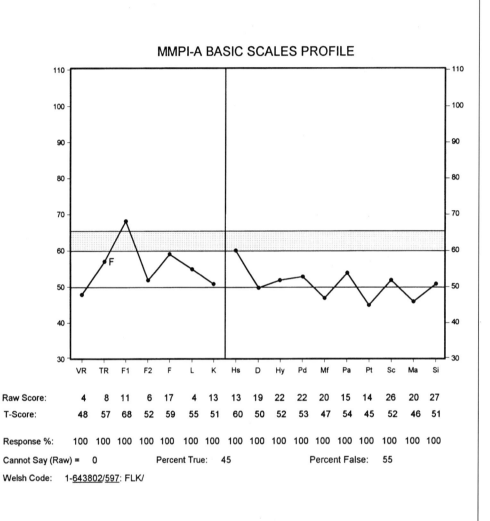

MMPI-A BASIC SCALES PROFILE

	VR	TR	F1	F2	F	L	K	Hs	D	Hy	Pd	Mf	Pa	Pt	Sc	Ma	Si
Raw Score:	4	8	11	6	17	4	13	13	19	22	22	20	15	14	26	20	27
T-Score:	48	57	68	52	59	55	51	60	50	52	53	47	54	45	52	46	51
Response %:	100	100	100	100	100	100	100	100	100	100	100	100	100	100	100	100	100

Cannot Say (Raw) =   0   Percent True: 45   Percent False: 55

Welsh Code: 1-643802/597: FLK/

CASE 1
"ANTHONY"

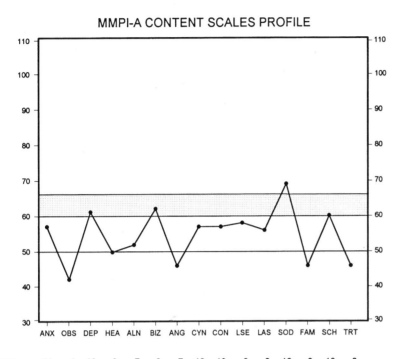

MMPI-A CONTENT SCALES PROFILE

	ANX	OBS	DEP	HEA	ALN	BIZ	ANG	CYN	CON	LSE	LAS	SOD	FAM	SCH	TRT
Raw Score:	11	4	13	8	7	8	7	16	13	8	8	16	9	10	8
T-Score:	57	42	61	50	52	62	46	57	57	58	56	69	46	60	46
Response %:	100	100	100	100	100	100	100	100	100	100	100	100	100	100	100

CASE 1
"ANTHONY"

MMPI-A
ID 1

Extended Score Report
Page 4

SUPPLEMENTARY SCORE REPORT

	Raw Score	T Score	Resp %
MacAndrew Alcoholism-Revised (MAC-R)	17	41	100
Alcohol/Drug Problem Acknowledgement (ACK)	2	42	100
Alcohol/Drug Problem Proneness (PRO)	12	40	100
Immaturity Scale (IMM)	22	64	100
Anxiety (A)	12	46	100
Repression (R)	14	51	100

Depression Subscales (Harris-Lingoes)

	Raw Score	T Score	Resp %
Subjective Depression (D1)	8	49	100
Psychomotor Retardation (D2)	3	41	100
Physical Malfunctioning (D3)	4	55	100
Mental Dullness (D4)	2	43	100
Brooding (D5)	4	56	100

Hysteria Subscales (Harris-Lingoes)

	Raw Score	T Score	Resp %
Denial of Social Anxiety (Hy1)	4	55	100
Need for Affection (Hy2)	4	46	100
Lassitude-Malaise (Hy3)	5	54	100
Somatic Complaints (Hy4)	4	50	100
Inhibition of Aggression (Hy5)	3	51	100

Psychopathic Deviate Subscales (Harris-Lingoes)

	Raw Score	T Score	Resp %
Familial Discord (Pd1)	1	37	100
Authority Problems (Pd2)	5	60	100
Social Imperturbability (Pd3)	3	48	100
Social Alienation (Pd4)	4	46	100
Self-Alienation (Pd5)	4	49	100

Paranoia Subscales (Harris-Lingoes)

	Raw Score	T Score	Resp %
Persecutory Ideas (Pa1)	8	64	100
Poignancy (Pa2)	2	42	100
Naivete (Pa3)	3	45	100

Schizophrenia Subscales (Harris-Lingoes)

Social Alienation (Sc1)	9	59	100
Emotional Alienation (Sc2)	3	54	100
Lack of Ego Mastery, Cognitive (Sc3)	3	50	100
Lack of Ego Mastery, Conative (Sc4)	4	50	100
Lack of Ego Mastery, Defective Inhibition (Sc5)	3	48	100
Bizarre Sensory Experiences (Sc6)	3	44	100

Hypomania Subscales (Harris-Lingoes)

Amorality (Ma1)	5	66	100
Psychomotor Acceleration (Ma2)	5	43	100
Imperturbability (Ma3)	4	55	100
Ego Inflation (Ma4)	3	42	100

Social Introversion Subscales (Ben-Porath, Hostetler, Butcher, & Graham)

Shyness / Self-Consciousness (Si1)	5	46	100
Social Avoidance (Si2)	7	72	100
Alienation--Self and Others (Si3)	6	45	100

Uniform T scores are used for Hs, D, Hy, Pd, Pa, Pt, Sc, Ma, and the Content Scales; all other MMPI-A scales use linear T scores.

End of Report

CASE 1
"ANTHONY"

SUGGESTED ITEMS FOR FOLLOW-UP

SUICIDAL BEHAVIORS

283. Most of the time I wish I were dead. (T)

SUICIDAL BEHAVIORS

CASE 2
"BRENDA"

A YOUNGSTER CRIES FOR HELP

BACKGROUND

Brenda is a 16-year-old, Caucasian female who was seen for an outpatient diagnostic psychological evaluation. She had been placed in the custody of the local county children's services agency as a result of severe parent/child conflict and unruly behavior. In the following five months, she had a series of out of home placements. She was referred for psychological evaluation because of her behavior as well as reports of current depression and a history of several suicide attempts.

Brenda's parents married when they were 18 years old and were divorced during her first year of life. Her parents lived apart for one year and then the father moved back into the house for nine years before they separated again. They remarried shortly before the time of this evaluation. The mother was described by Brenda as being "uptight and controlling" and as having been adopted by alcoholic parents at the age of 11 months. Brenda stated that she "hates her mother." At the time of the evaluation, it was reported that the mother remained the primary decision-maker in the family. Brenda's father was described by her as "easygoing." He is the youngest of four children and the family was described

as close. However, his mother died of a severe illness when he was nine years old and he was raised by his two sisters. His father died one year before the evaluation, and this reportedly continued to have a profound effect upon him. He was involved with Brenda but played a generally passive role in the family. Brenda's sister is two years older and was described by her as "perfect . . . totally different from me." At the time of the assessment the sister was attending college and was reported to be favored by the mother.

Brenda's mother's pregnancy and delivery of Brenda were reported to be without complications and Brenda achieved developmental milestones appropriately. She was described as a happy child but one who tested limits constantly. The first reports of negative behavior occurred in preschool when Brenda was seen as oppositional. In spite of obtaining passing grades, her mother requested that she be held back in the fourth grade because she was struggling academically and her mother did not approve of her choice of friends. Considerable behavioral problems were seen at the onset of puberty. Brenda reportedly first felt suicidal in the fifth grade at age 11 and in the sixth grade she overdosed on Tylenol and cut her wrists. She stated that the reason that she felt suicidal was the controlling nature of her mother. She made her first suicide attempt jointly with a friend who was also experiencing family conflict. One year later, she made another suicide attempt by overdose in school. She was admitted to an inpatient unit for three weeks and then returned home. Shortly thereafter, she again became depressed and oppositional and was readmitted to the hospital. Before the second hospitalization, she was described as showing considerable oppositional behavior and as lying, stealing, and being vindictive. The record indicated that three of her friends had also taken overdoses in the preceding three weeks. After the last hospitalization, Brenda lived with her father but was generally unsupervised. She then began dating a 23–year–old man as well as becoming highly sexually active and abusing marijuana, some of which she obtained from her father. Her acting out escalated to the point that she was placed in emergency shelter care on three occasions. At the time of the evaluation, she was living with a friend and had dropped out of high school. There was no reported history of physical or sexual abuse.

During this period, she episodically participated in outpatient care that included individual, family, and group counseling. Brenda was prescribed Prozac, an antidepressant, but refused to take the medication.

In her clinical interview, Brenda presented as a slightly overweight adolescent who was dressed casually but neatly. There were no overt indications of gross or fine motor dysfunctions. Her gait and posture were nonremarkable. Her speech was normal in tone, pacing, and volume. She did not evidence loosening of associations, flight of ideas or tangentiality. Her eye contact was direct. She was quite cooperative with the evaluation and engaged easily with the examiner. Her mood was seen as depressed, and her affect was expressive and appropriate to this mood. She denied experiencing, and there were no indications of, hallucinations, delusions, or organized paranoid

ideation. She acknowledged feeling depressed and complained of low mood, fatigue, low motivation, hypersomnia, and social withdrawal. She also reported that she felt "empty, angry, irritable, and disinterested in activities," with feelings of hopelessness and worthlessness. She also stated that she could get quite depressed about her weight, "and stop eating for at least a week, I think about my weight every day." It was also noted that the mother was quite overweight and tended to be highly critical concerning the client's weight. Brenda stated that she experiences mood shifts and feels "generally quite moody." She described herself as having a poor attitude, "I don't care about anything and I have no idea why I feel like this, I get these moods about four times a day." When she experiences these moods, which last for varying periods of time, she stated that she wants to verbally attack others and destroy things. She was oriented to time, place, and person. Her insight and judgment were assessed as nonremarkable.

Brenda was administered a battery of tests including the MMPI–A, the WISC–III, the Incomplete Sentences Blank, and the Children's Depression Inventory. She was found to have a full scale IQ of 86, a performance score of 99, and a verbal score of 78. This intelligence test score was seen as a possible underestimation of her abilities owing to her current emotional distress and psychosocial stressors. On the ISB, she focussed primarily on positive statements about her boyfriend and negative comments about her mother, and described herself as being generally quite angry. On the CDI, she generated a clinically significant elevation of 82, with her highest scores on the subtests of negative mood and ineffectiveness. However, all the subtests were elevated in the clinically significant range.

MMPI–A INTERPRETATION
Profile Validity

Brenda's scores on the MMPI–A validity scales raise questions regarding the validity of her profile. She produced elevated scores on F and its two subscales, F_1 and F_2. Her level of elevation on these scales indicates that Brenda provided a relatively large number of deviant responses to the MMPI–A items. There are three, non–mutually exclusive reasons for elevation on the MMPI–A F scales: (a) random responding, (b) severe psychological problems, and (c) exaggeration or faking.

The first possibility, random responding, is counter–indicated by Brenda's below average T score on VRIN, the MMPI–A random response indicator. The second possibility, severe psychological problems, is consistent with the background information and clinical observations made during the evaluation. Thus, the possibility of fabrication of psychological problems is not indicated in this case. Examination of Brenda's clinical and content scale profiles indicates a diffuse pattern of elevation. This, coupled with the level of elevation on F, indicates that the most likely cause of her pattern of scores is genuine psychological problems, the magnitude of which may have been somewhat exaggerated in a test approach that has traditionally been labeled a "cry for help."

In sum, Brenda's scores on the MMPI–A validity scales indicate that she produced a valid MMPI–A profile. She provided a consistent set of responses to the test items. However, she may have exaggerated in describing some of her problems in an attempt to draw attention to her psychological distress.

Current Level of Adjustment

Brenda's MMPI–A profile indicates that she is experiencing considerable psychological distress and turmoil at this time, and that she likely feels overwhelmed by her current psychological difficulties. There are numerous indications of severe distress in Brenda's profile. The level of the F elevation indicates that she is reporting a large number of problems in different areas of her life. She produced clinically elevated scores on seven of the eight original clinical scales and on all but two of the content scales. Among

the clinical scales she produced her most elevated score on Scale 2, which is one of the clinical scales most highly correlated with current level of maladjustment. She also produced highly elevated scores on Scales 7 and 8, which are additional indicators of current level of distress.

Symptoms and Traits

Brenda's most elevated score on the clinical profile is on Scale 2. This indicates that she is likely experiencing a very depressed mood and that she is likely very pessimistic about her future. She is likely to be very self–critical and to experience guilt over her perceived shortcomings. She may also be experiencing a high degree of anxiety and she may express various somatic concerns. Adolescents in clinical settings who produce elevated scores on this scale tend to be shy, timid, and socially withdrawn. Adolescent girls also are likely to have eating problems. Examination of the Harris and Lingoes subscales for Scale 2 does not indicate that Brenda's elevation on this scale stems from any particular content area. As in any case where the MMPI–A indicates a strong likelihood of depression, the possibility of suicidal ideation needs to be considered. In this case, examination of the Suggested Items for Follow–up indicates that Brenda has endorsed two suicidal items. Thus, an immediate suicide assessment is indicated. In Brenda's case we know from her background that she has made several suicide attempts, highlighting further the need for a thorough assessment of her current risk for suicide.

Brenda produced secondary elevations on several other clinical scales. Her elevation on Scale 1 indicates further that she is somewhat preoccupied with physical health concerns at this time. Examination of her scores on the relevant Harris and Lingoes subscales indicates that Brenda's elevation on Scale 3 stems primarily from complaints of feeling weak, tired, and generally dysphoric. Brenda's elevation on Scale 4 indicates that she is prone toward acting-out behaviors, that she resents authority figures, and that she is likely to have had academic and behavioral problems in school. Her score on this scale also indicates that Brenda may have considerable problems with her family and that she is at risk for developing substance-use problems.

Given her pattern of scores on the subscales for Scale 6, Brenda's elevation on this scale seems to stem primarily from a belief that she is often criticized without cause and from a hypersensitivity to criticism. Brenda's elevation on Scale 7 is consistent with the view that she is experiencing considerable psychological distress and turmoil at this time. It indicates further the strong possibility that Brenda has a very poor self–image and that she tends to set very high goals for herself and to become very self–critical when she does not accomplish these goals.

Brenda's elevation on Scale 8 suggests the *possibility* that she may be experiencing some psychotic symptoms. However, her relatively low score on the Bizarre Sensory Experiences subscale and her relatively low score on the content scale Adolescent Bizarre Mentation (A–biz) counterindicate this interpretation. Thus, her elevated score on Scale 8 is consistent with other indications on Brenda's MMPI–A profile that she is experiencing a great deal of psychological turmoil and upheaval at this time. Finally, Brenda's elevated score on Scale 0 indicates that she tends to be shy and timid around others and is uncomfortable in social situations.

Brenda's scores on the MMPI–A content scales are consistent with what has already been observed about her clinical scale scores. These scales highlight that one of Brenda's most significant areas of concern is her very low self-esteem and that she also reports a great deal of family conflict and dysfunction. She tends to feel very alienated from others and has no confidence in her ability to solve her problems on her own. She also acknowledges having considerable difficulties in school and having had problems controlling her anger. In light of the prominent elevation she generated on most of the content scales,

Brenda's relatively low score on Adolescent Negative Treatment Indicators (A–trt) can be viewed as a positive indication that she has not given up hope of being helped.

In sum, Brenda's scores on the MMPI–A indicate that she is feeling very depressed and anxious at this time. She has very low self–confidence and tends to be very self–critical and self–punitive. Brenda likely has very high and unrealistic expectations for herself and she tends to "set up" situations in which she will fail to live up to these expectations. When this happens, she tends to become very sullen and angry. She is also at substantial risk for suicidal ideation and behavior. Brenda tends to feel very uncomfortable around others, and she views her family as a source of difficulty rather than as a place to turn for support. There are a few positive indications in Brenda's MMPI–A profile. These include her relatively low score on A–trt, her substantial level of current psychological distress, and her "cry for help" approach to the testing, all of which indicate that Brenda may currently be motivated to receive psychological intervention.

Diagnostic Suggestions

As summarized in the description of Brenda's background, two primary concerns led to this evaluation: her depression and her acting-out behavior. Brenda's MMPI–A profile is clearly consistent with the diagnosis of a depressive disorder, and her level of depression and distress suggests the possibility of a major depressive episode. Regarding her acting-out behavior, although Brenda's profile is consistent with a diagnosis of conduct or oppositional disorder, her profile indicates that Brenda's acting-out behavior is currently secondary to her more severe emotional problems and may possibly be a product of these problems rather than a manifestation of an underlying personality disorder. Finally, Brenda's scores on the MMPI–A supplementary scales indicate that she is at substantial risk for developing a substance-use problem, although she does not acknowledge having such a problem at this time. She produced a very high score on the Alcohol/Drug Problem Proneness (PRO) scale, which indicates that Brenda has a number of personality characteristics and behavioral tendencies that place her at substantial risk for developing an alcohol and/or drug problem. She may be particularly susceptible to the negative influence of peers in this respect. She also produced an elevated score on the Revised MacAndrew (MAC–R) scale, further substantiating Brenda's vulnerability to problems in this area. However, it should be emphasized that these scores do not, in themselves, indicate that Brenda actually has an alcohol or drug problem. But they do indicate the presence of substantial risk in this area.

Treatment Recommendations

Brenda's MMPI–A profile indicates that initial treatment efforts should focus on addressing her depression and anxiety. The potential benefits of medication should be considered and a careful evaluation of her potential for suicide should be conducted. In addition to addressing these acute issues, Brenda is a good candidate for individual therapy to focus on her mood symptoms as well as on her very low self–esteem and her tendency to set unrealistic goals and expectations for herself. In light of the considerable family turmoil suggested by her profile, the possibility of family therapy should also be explored. Finally, a careful evaluation of Brenda's potential for developing alcohol and drug problems is indicated.

OUTCOME

Brenda received a diagnosis of Major Depressive Disorder, Recurrent, without psychotic features; Conduct Disorder, mild; Parent Child Relational Problems and R/O Learning Disorder, NOS. Treatment interventions recommended for this youth included individual therapy, particularly a supportive approach, psychiatric referral for potential medication, family therapy, ongoing evaluation for presence of suicidal thoughts or behaviors, and psycho–educational, vocational evaluations and interventions.

MMPI-A*

Extended Score Report

ID Number 2

Brenda

Female

Age 16

10/18/94

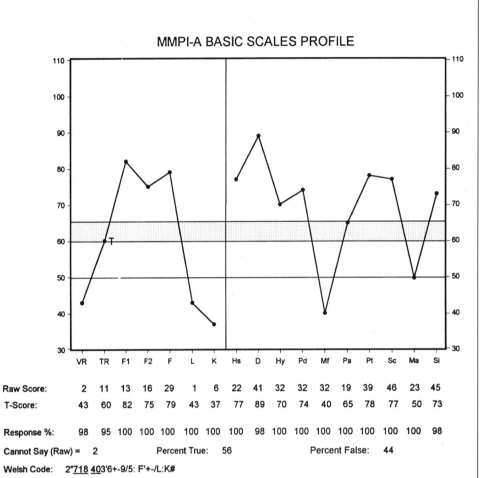

MMPI-A BASIC SCALES PROFILE

	VR	TR	F1	F2	F	L	K	Hs	D	Hy	Pd	Mf	Pa	Pt	Sc	Ma	Si
Raw Score:	2	11	13	16	29	1	6	22	41	32	32	32	19	39	46	23	45
T-Score:	43	60	82	75	79	43	37	77	89	70	74	40	65	78	77	50	73
Response %:	98	95	100	100	100	100	100	100	98	100	100	100	100	100	100	100	98

Cannot Say (Raw) = 2   Percent True: 56   Percent False: 44

Welsh Code: 2"718 403'6+-9/5: F'+-/L:K#

CASE 2
"BRENDA"

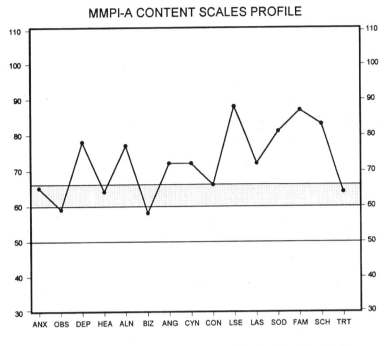

MMPI-A CONTENT SCALES PROFILE

	ANX	OBS	DEP	HEA	ALN	BIZ	ANG	CYN	CON	LSE	LAS	SOD	FAM	SCH	TRT
Raw Score:	15	11	22	17	14	7	14	20	14	17	11	19	28	15	15
T-Score:	65	59	78	64	77	58	72	72	66	88	72	81	87	83	64
Response %:	100	100	96	100	100	100	100	100	100	100	94	100	100	100	96

SUPPLEMENTARY SCORE REPORT

	Raw Score	T Score	Resp %
MacAndrew Alcoholism-Revised (MAC-R)	26	65	100
Alcohol/Drug Problem Acknowledgement (ACK)	5	56	100
Alcohol/Drug Problem Proneness (PRO)	31	84	100
Immaturity Scale (IMM)	26	73	98
Anxiety (A)	27	63	100
Repression (R)	19	66	100

Depression Subscales (Harris-Lingoes)

	Raw Score	T Score	Resp %
Subjective Depression (D1)	27	87	97
Psychomotor Retardation (D2)	10	78	100
Physical Malfunctioning (D3)	8	77	100
Mental Dullness (D4)	14	89	93
Brooding (D5)	8	70	90

Hysteria Subscales (Harris-Lingoes)

	Raw Score	T Score	Resp %
Denial of Social Anxiety (Hy1)	1	37	100
Need for Affection (Hy2)	2	38	100
Lassitude-Malaise (Hy3)	15	87	100
Somatic Complaints (Hy4)	11	70	100
Inhibition of Aggression (Hy5)	1	35	100

Psychopathic Deviate Subscales (Harris-Lingoes)

	Raw Score	T Score	Resp %
Familial Discord (Pd1)	7	66	100
Authority Problems (Pd2)	5	65	100
Social Imperturbability (Pd3)	0	30	100
Social Alienation (Pd4)	6	53	100
Self-Alienation (Pd5)	11	75	100

Paranoia Subscales (Harris-Lingoes)

	Raw Score	T Score	Resp %
Persecutory Ideas (Pa1)	6	57	100
Poignancy (Pa2)	8	73	100
Naivete (Pa3)	1	36	100

MMPI-A
ID 2

Extended Score Report
Page 5

CASE 2
"BRENDA"

Schizophrenia Subscales (Harris-Lingoes)

Social Alienation (Sc1)	15	76	100
Emotional Alienation (Sc2)	6	70	100
Lack of Ego Mastery, Cognitive (Sc3)	8	71	100
Lack of Ego Mastery, Conative (Sc4)	10	71	100
Lack of Ego Mastery, Defective Inhibition (Sc5)	5	54	100
Bizarre Sensory Experiences (Sc6)	9	60	100

Hypomania Subscales (Harris-Lingoes)

Amorality (Ma1)	3	55	100
Psychomotor Acceleration (Ma2)	6	44	100
Imperturbability (Ma3)	1	37	100
Ego Inflation (Ma4)	5	52	100

Social Introversion Subscales (Ben-Porath, Hostetler, Butcher, & Graham)

Shyness / Self-Consciousness (Si1)	10	62	100
Social Avoidance (Si2)	8	83	100
Alienation--Self and Others (Si3)	12	60	94

Uniform T scores are used for Hs, D, Hy, Pd, Pa, Pt, Sc, Ma, and the Content Scales; all other MMPI-A scales use linear T scores.

OMITTED ITEMS

The following items were omitted by the client. It may be helpful to discuss these item omissions with this individual to determine the reason for non-compliance with test instructions.

27. I shrink from facing a crisis or difficulty.
71. I usually feel that life is worthwhile.

End of Report

SUGGESTED ITEMS FOR FOLLOW-UP

ALCOHOL/DRUG PROBLEMS

161. I have had periods in which I carried on activities without knowing later what I had been doing. (T)

467. I enjoy using marijuana. (T)

SUICIDAL BEHAVIORS

177. I sometimes think about killing myself. (T)

283. Most of the time I wish I were dead. (T)

FAMILY PROBLEMS

440. I have spent nights away from home when my parents did not know where I was. (T)

460. I have never run away from home. (F)

CASE 3
"CASEY"

A GUARDED, ANGRY YOUNGSTER
LACKING IN INSIGHT

BACKGROUND

Casey is a 16-year-old, Caucasian male evaluated on an outpatient basis. He had been brought for evaluation by his father because he reacted with uncontrollable rage when limits were placed upon him. It was alleged that he had threatened to cut off his sister's fingers with an ax. He is reported to have frequent, wide mood swings, dysphoria, oppositional behavior, and a history of Polysubstance abuse. There is a history of suicidal and homicidal ideation, and it is reported that he once brought a gun and switchblade into his home. It is also reported that he has stolen a large amount of money from his father.

Casey is the older of two children born to an intact family. His mother's pregnancy and his birth were non-remarkable. Casey achieved his developmental milestones normally. There is no history of serious childhood injury, head trauma, coma, or major surgeries. He was described as being a difficult child and as having frequent temper tantrums. He demonstrated oppositional and aggressive behavior since elementary school. There is no documented history of abuse. There is, as well, no documented history of mental illness or criminal justice system involvement in his family.

During his clinical interview, Casey was observed to be dressed in street clothes which were neat, clean, and appropriate to the current season. His hygiene and grooming were adequate. His gait and posture were non-remarkable, and there were no overt indications of gross or fine motor dysfunction. His speech was normal in tone, pacing, and volume. His verbalizations were coherent, goal-directed, and without indications of loosening of associations, flight of ideas, or tangentiality. His attention span was adequate and he was not distractible. His manner of social interaction was intense and controlling.

Casey presented an appropriate affect to a stated neutral mood. He denied experiencing, and there were no overt indications of, hallucinations, delusions, or organized paranoid ideation. He reported periods of depression with episodic suicidal ideation, as well as some nonspecific thoughts of harming others. He specifically denied present intent to harm himself or anyone else. He stated that the incident with the gun was "a mistake." He denied current disturbances in his sleep, health, or appetite. He did appear to be anhedonic. There were no current clinical indications of significant anxiety, phobias, obsessions, or compulsions. He was oriented to time, place, and person. His long-term, short-term, and immediate recall functions were intact. He could interpret proverbs and identify similarities between related objects. His insight and judgment appeared to be below age expectations.

MMPI–A INTERPRETATION
Profile Validity

Casey's scores on the MMPI–A validity scales do not raise any substantial concerns regarding profile validity. He responded to all of the test items and appeared to do so in a relatively straightforward manner. His scores on the MMPI–A consistency scales indicate that Casey was careful not to contradict himself and that he produced a smaller than average number of deviant responses. This pattern is somewhat inconsistent with the nature of the referral, which included descriptions of very deviant behavior.

Casey's score on the K validity scale approaches the cutoff for clinically meaningful elevation, indicating a tendency on his part toward defensiveness. Such a pattern is less common in adolescents than it is in adults, and it is particularly uncommon in adolescents who are seen in clinical settings. Adolescents in clinical settings who produce this level of elevation on K are unwilling to admit having psychological problems, and they tend to deny any need for treatment or assistance. They often hide behind a facade of adequate coping and adjustment.

In the relatively infrequent cases where adolescents generate defensive MMPI–A profiles, they are not very likely to produce any elevation on the content scales. However, sometimes it is informative to examine the content scales to determine whether there are any areas about which the adolescent is particularly reluctant to report difficulties. An examination of Casey's MMPI–A profile indicates that there were two areas of functioning where he reported considerably fewer difficulties than the "average" adolescent in a nonclinical setting: anger problems and social discomfort.

Although Casey's low scores on the Adolescent Anger (A–ang) and Adolescent Social Discomfort (A-sod) scales can by no means be viewed as positive indicators that he has difficulties in these areas, these scores do raise the possibility that Casey may be particularly reluctant to discuss any difficulties he might have with anger control and social relationships.

Overall, Casey produced a valid MMPI–A profile. However, his approach to the test was somewhat defensive and he appeared to be particularly reluctant to acknowledge any difficulties in the areas of anger control and social relationships.

Current Level of Adjustment

Casey's MMPI–A profile indicates that he is not experiencing psychological distress at this time. However, he is reporting some adjustment difficulties. The negative slope of his MMPI–A profile indicates a "neurotic" pattern of maladjustment. Casey's problems are not likely to cause him significant debilitation, but they may be manifested in occasional periods of greater difficulty.

Symptoms and Traits

Casey produced a very prominent elevation on MMPI–A clinical Scale 3. This is a very unusual elevation for adolescents in general, and boys in particular. His score on this scale suggests that Casey tends to be immature, self–centered, and demanding of attention. He enjoys being the center of attention and becomes frustrated when he believes that he is not receiving sufficient attention and praise. His elevation on this scale suggests further that Casey tends to respond to stress by developing, or complaining of, physical health concerns. He may also be feeling somewhat depressed at this time, and he may engage in some suicidal ideation. He tends to deny having any psychological problems.

Casey also produced a clinically elevated score on Scale 1. This elevation indicates further that Casey tends to be preoccupied with physical health concerns. It also suggests the possibility that in spite of his bold, secure, facade Casey may harbor considerable fears and insecurities. This elevation also suggests that Casey tends to be self–centered, demanding, and attention–seeking. Casey's elevation on Scale 4 indicates that he is prone toward acting-out behavior. His scores on the subscales of this scale indicate that Casey reports experiencing some family problems and that he tends to feel somewhat alienated from his own thoughts and feelings.

Casey's moderately elevated score on Scale 2 suggests that he may be experiencing some depression at this time. However, his pattern of scores on Scales 1, 2, and 3 indicates that Casey is likely to downplay the emotional component of his problems and focus on somatic complaints.

Casey produced a *very* low score on Scale 0. This score indicates that Casey presents himself as being very open and outgoing and having far fewer social inhibitions than most other adolescents. However, given Casey's scores on the other clinical scales, particularly on Scale 3, it would appear that Casey's presentation of social poise may be a facade designed to mask deep–rooted anxieties and inhibitions.

Overall, his MMPI–A profile indicates that Casey tends to be immature and self–centered, that he tends to deny or minimize psychological problems, and that he tends to develop or perceive somatic problems when he experiences stress or distress. Casey is likely to have limited insight into his own situation and behavior. Although he attempts to portray himself as a confident young man who is free of any major concerns, Casey appears to harbor significant fears and insecurities to which he may respond by occasional outbursts of anger and frustration. He has some acting-out tendencies and apparently has conflicts with members of his family.

Diagnostic Suggestions

Casey's MMPI–A profile suggests a number of diagnostic possibilities. Because of the indications of acting-out tendencies, the possibility of a conduct disorder should be considered. The possibility of a personality disorder with histrionic and narcissistic features is indicated by Casey's apparent strong need for attention and admiration, and the possibility that he is prone to over–react with considerable anger in response to seemingly minor provocation.

Casey's scores on the MMPI–A substance-use scales indicate that he is at risk for developing alcohol and/or drug problems. His score on the Alcohol/Drug Problem Proneness (PRO) scale suggests that Casey possesses certain personality characteristics that place him at risk for developing alcohol or drug problems. He may be particularly vulnerable to the negative influences of peers in this area. His score on the Revised MacAndrew (MAC–R) scale supports further the indication that Casey possesses personality characteristics that place him at risk for substance abuse. His relatively low score on the Alcohol/Drug Problem Acknowledgment (ACK) scale, indicates that Casey does not acknowledge many difficulties in this area at this time. However, inspection of his responses to the list of Suggested Items for Follow–up indicates that Casey does acknowledge having used marijuana.

Treatment Recommendations

Casey's overall defensive pattern, his tendency to deny and cover up problems, and his general lack of insight do not bode well for him in any potential psychological treatment program. His MMPI–A profile suggests that Casey is not likely to comply with traditional insight–oriented psychotherapy. He may be better served by the development of a behavioral modification and anger-management program with very specific and realistic goals. A careful screening for substance-abuse problems should be conducted. Because of family conflict indicated in Casey's MMPI–A profile, the possibility of family therapy should be explored. Further information on the nature of conflict in Casey's family is needed to determine the focus of any plan for family therapy.

OUTCOME

Casey received a diagnosis of Conduct Disorder, Dysthymia and Histrionic Personality Traits. It was recommended that he not return home, and he was placed in a treatment foster home where he also received individual, cognitive behavioral therapy, anger-management and family therapy.

MMPI-A*

Extended Score Report

ID Number 3

Casey

Male

Age 16

2/15/94

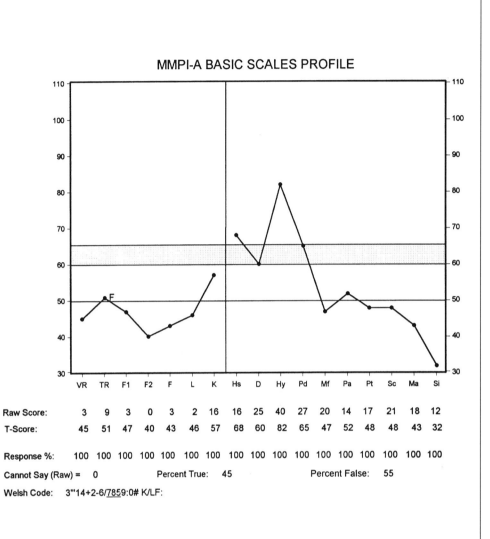

MMPI-A BASIC SCALES PROFILE

	VR	TR	F1	F2	F	L	K	Hs	D	Hy	Pd	Mf	Pa	Pt	Sc	Ma	Si
Raw Score:	3	9	3	0	3	2	16	16	25	40	27	20	14	17	21	18	12
T-Score:	45	51	47	40	43	46	57	68	60	82	65	47	52	48	48	43	32
Response %:	100	100	100	100	100	100	100	100	100	100	100	100	100	100	100	100	100

Cannot Say (Raw) =   0   Percent True: 45   Percent False: 55

Welsh Code: 3'''14+2-6/7859:0# K/LF:

CASE 3
"CASEY"

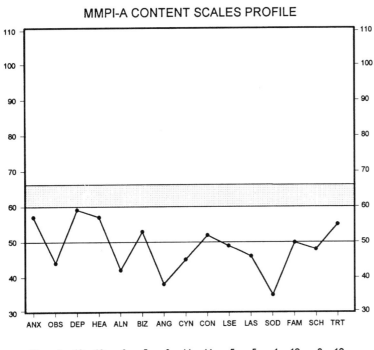

MMPI-A CONTENT SCALES PROFILE

	ANX	OBS	DEP	HEA	ALN	BIZ	ANG	CYN	CON	LSE	LAS	SOD	FAM	SCH	TRT
Raw Score:	11	5	12	13	3	5	3	11	11	5	5	1	12	6	12
T-Score:	57	44	59	57	42	53	38	45	52	49	46	35	50	48	55
Response %:	100	100	100	100	100	100	100	100	100	100	100	100	100	100	100

SUPPLEMENTARY SCORE REPORT

	Raw Score	T Score	Resp %
MacAndrew Alcoholism-Revised (MAC-R)	26	61	100
Alcohol/Drug Problem Acknowledgement (ACK)	3	46	100
Alcohol/Drug Problem Proneness (PRO)	23	65	100
Immaturity Scale (IMM)	11	46	100
Anxiety (A)	15	51	100
Repression (R)	13	49	100

Depression Subscales (Harris-Lingoes)

Subjective Depression (D1)	15	65	100
Psychomotor Retardation (D2)	9	71	100
Physical Malfunctioning (D3)	3	48	100
Mental Dullness (D4)	6	60	100
Brooding (D5)	4	56	100

Hysteria Subscales (Harris-Lingoes)

Denial of Social Anxiety (Hy1)	5	61	100
Need for Affection (Hy2)	9	67	100
Lassitude-Malaise (Hy3)	12	81	100
Somatic Complaints (Hy4)	8	64	100
Inhibition of Aggression (Hy5)	4	59	100

Psychopathic Deviate Subscales (Harris-Lingoes)

Familial Discord (Pd1)	6	64	100
Authority Problems (Pd2)	3	48	100
Social Imperturbability (Pd3)	4	54	100
Social Alienation (Pd4)	6	55	100
Self-Alienation (Pd5)	10	73	100

Paranoia Subscales (Harris-Lingoes)

Persecutory Ideas (Pa1)	3	46	100
Poignancy (Pa2)	4	55	100
Naivete (Pa3)	7	66	100

Schizophrenia Subscales (Harris-Lingoes)

Social Alienation (Sc1)	3	40	100
Emotional Alienation (Sc2)	3	54	100
Lack of Ego Mastery, Cognitive (Sc3)	5	59	100
Lack of Ego Mastery, Conative (Sc4)	7	61	100
Lack of Ego Mastery, Defective Inhibition (Sc5)	3	48	100
Bizarre Sensory Experiences (Sc6)	2	41	100

Hypomania Subscales (Harris-Lingoes)

Amorality (Ma1)	4	59	100
Psychomotor Acceleration (Ma2)	7	52	100
Imperturbability (Ma3)	3	49	100
Ego Inflation (Ma4)	3	42	100

Social Introversion Subscales (Ben-Porath, Hostetler, Butcher, & Graham)

Shyness / Self-Consciousness (Si1)	1	33	100
Social Avoidance (Si2)	0	38	100
Alienation--Self and Others (Si3)	6	45	100

Uniform T scores are used for Hs, D, Hy, Pd, Pa, Pt, Sc, Ma, and the Content Scales; all other MMPI-A scales use linear T scores.

End of Report

SUGGESTED ITEMS FOR FOLLOW-UP

ALCOHOL/DRUG PROBLEMS

467. I enjoy using marijuana. (T)

CASE 4
"DEBBIE"

A MIXED PRESENTATION OF
SEVERE ANXIETY AND DEPRESSION

BACKGROUND

Debbie is a 15-year-old, Caucasian female who was referred for psychological consultation to aid in differential diagnosis and outpatient treatment planning. Her presenting problems at the time of assessment included disabling migraine headaches, severe anxiety, and depression thought to be centered around conflicts about being in school. It was reported that primarily because of the severity of her symptoms and her fear of losing control, she was removed from her high school two months before the evaluation and was receiving home instruction.

Debbie was raised by her maternal grandmother since early childhood. Her biological parents were never married, and she saw her father for the first time only three years before the evaluation. She continues to have only minimal contact with him and feels severely rejected by him. Debbie's biological mother was 15 years old when she gave birth to the client. She is now married to a man who is reported to be an alcoholic. It is also reported that he is verbally and physically abusive and that he has injured the mother to the degree that she has had to receive hospital treatment for her injuries. It is also reported that

Debbie's mother has a problem with drinking as well as significant episodes of depression. In the past year, Debbie has had to intervene twice to prevent her mother from committing suicide. She would sometimes visit her mother, but these visits have ceased owing to the violence against the mother by the stepfather.

Her mother is reported to have had a normal pregnancy and Debbie's delivery was also normal. She achieved developmental milestones appropriately. She was described as being a shy and anxious child. There is no apparent history of physical or sexual abuse. She has no other siblings. She did have some friends in elementary school and has always earned very good grades. She was an honor student in middle school but appeared to begin to lose interest at that time. Her symptoms have increased in severity and intensity over the past two years. She reported that on the days that she attended school, she was in "severe agony." She described feelings of self-consciousness, sweaty palms, nausea, dizziness, and depersonalization. These symptoms became debilitating for her, and her grandmother would often pick her up at school and take her home. Despite her absence from school, Debbie continues to maintain relationships with her school friends. She does things socially with them and goes to the mall and movies. At such times, she reports that she does have the physical symptoms but that they are manageable for her.

Her grandmother expressed considerable concern that Debbie would not graduate from high school with her peers. She also indicated worry that Debbie will not be able to support herself as an adult. In the initial interview, she turned to Debbie and warned her that she "won't always be around to support" her and that she needs to complete school to be self-sufficient. Debbie fairly quickly admitted that she did not plan to return to school but wanted to be tutored at home for the remainder of her school years.

In clinical interview, Debbie presented as an attractive female who appeared to be about her stated age. Her clothing was neat, clean, stylish, and appropriate to the season. Her hygiene and grooming were excellent. Her gait and posture were nonremarkable and there were no overt indications of gross or fine motor dysfunctions. Her speech was normal in tone, somewhat slowed in pacing and lowered in volume. There were no indications of loosening of associations, flight of ideas, or tangentiality. Her attention span was adequate and her level of psychomotor activity was nonremarkable. Interpersonally, she seemed to be hesitant, almost conflictual about interacting with the examiner. Debbie presented with an appropriate affect to a stated mildly anxious and depressed mood. She denied experiencing, and there were no current indications of, hallucinations, delusions, or organized paranoid ideation.

Debbie reported that she has been quite frightened of being around people for as long as she can remember. She indicated that she wants to have social contact but is afraid of what people might think about her. She indicated that she has stayed up all night worrying about school but that she currently sleeps through the night. She denied disturbances in her appetite. She also complained of intrusive thoughts of

worry about school. These thoughts interfere with her ability to concentrate. She also reported nonspecific feelings of dread and anxiety. On a subjective unit of disturbance scale, she reported her anxiety to be eight of a possible 10. She reported that during the past year she has had significant periods of depression, some of which were related to specific situations, others of which had no known cause. During such times, she feels overwhelmed, hopeless, and helpless. She sees herself as a chronically unhappy person. When she is significantly depressed, both her sleep and appetite are disturbed. At such times, she has episodic thoughts of killing herself by overdose. However, in the interview Debbie denied any present thoughts of suicide, had no active suicidal plan, and disclaimed any history of actually attempting to harm herself. As well, she denied any thoughts or history of harming others. Also, she did complain of obsessive worry about loss of control in school. Beyond her fears of school, no other phobias were elicited.

Debbie was oriented to time, place, and person. Her recall of digits was 7 forward and 5 reversed. She was able to state the last four presidents in the correct order and was able to recall three items from memory after distraction. She was able to correctly interpret proverbs and identify similarities between related objects. She had very limited insight into the possible psychological nature of her problems. Her judgment appeared to be age appropriate.

MMPI–A INTERPRETATION
Profile Validity

Debbie produced a valid MMPI–A profile. She responded to all the test items, and her scores on the consistency scales indicate that she provided a coherent and consistent set of responses. She has some elevation on F and the difference between F_1 and F_2 is inconsequential. Her elevation on F indicates that Debbie reported experiencing some psychological problems at this time. However, there are no indications of exaggeration or over–reporting of problems.

Overall, Debbie produced a valid MMPI–A profile. She responded to the test items in an honest and open manner, and the resulting MMPI–A profile should provide an accurate portrayal of her current psychological functioning.

Current Level of Adjustment

There are a number of indications in her profile that Debbie is presently experiencing substantial psychological distress. She produced clinically elevated scores on seven of the eight clinical scales and has a particularly elevated score on Scale 2, one of the MMPI–A scales that is most sensitive to current level of distress. She has an elevated score on the Welsh Anxiety (A) scale and numerous elevated scores among the MMPI–A content scales. This pattern of scores indicates that Debbie is experiencing considerable emotional discomfort at this time and that she may feel overwhelmed by her present difficulties.

Symptoms and Traits

Debbie's scores on the clinical scales indicate that she is very depressed at this time. Her elevation on Scale 2 and examination of her scores on the subscales for this scale indicate that she reports having a very dysphoric mood. She reports feeling very dissatisfied with her life and is likely experiencing feelings of hopelessness. Adolescents who produce elevated scores on this scale tend to be very self–critical and guilt–ridden. They lack confidence and are very pessimistic about their future. They also tend to become isolated socially because they are uncomfortable in the presence of others. Examination of the Suggested Items for Follow–up indicates that Debbie continues to express some suicidal ideation at this time.

Along with a very dysphoric mood, Debbie appears to be preoccupied with physical health concerns. Her elevation on Scales 1 and 3 indicates that she reports having a number of physical health problems. Her prominent elevation on Scale 3 indicates that Debbie is inclined to develop physical health problems or concerns in response to stress. She likely lacks insight into the connection between her physical symptoms and psychological problems. Debbie's combination of elevation on Scales 2 and 3 indicates that she is likely very over–controlled emotionally and that she is not likely to develop acting-out problems.

Debbie produced secondary elevations on a number of clinical scales. Her elevation on Scale 4 *might* suggest a tendency toward acting-out behaviors. However, examination of Debbie's scores on the subscales of Scale 4 indicates that the source of her elevation on this scale is its emotional alienation component, rather than acting-out tendencies. A similar examination of subscale score patterns shows that emotional alienation is also indicated by Debbie's moderately elevated score on Scale 8. Debbie's elevation on Scale 6 indicates that she is mistrusting of others and that she tends to be very sensitive to what she may perceive as criticism leveled at her by other individuals. Finally, Debbie's elevated score on Scale 0 provides further indication that she is very uncomfortable around people, that she feels very shy and self–conscious, and that Debbie tends to avoid situations where she might feel social discomfort.

Debbie's scores on the MMPI–A content scales provide further insight about how she perceives her problems. Her two highest elevations were on Adolescent Social Discomfort (A–sod) and Adolescent Anxiety (A–anx). Thus, Debbie reports feeling very uncomfortable in the presence of others and is very likely to avoid social situations. She is likely to be viewed by others as being socially withdrawn and depressed, and she is not likely to engage in acting-out behaviors. She likely feels very tense and anxious, and may fear losing control over her emotions.

Debbie produced several secondary elevations on the content scales that shed further light on her current functioning. Her elevated score on the Adolescent Obsessiveness (A–obs) scale indicates that Debbie is prone to obsessive rumination and that she likely has difficulties making decisions. Research indicates that adolescent girls tested in clinical settings who produce elevated scores on this scale are at increased risk for suicidal gestures. Her elevation on the Adolescent Depression (A–dep) content scale provides further indication that Debbie reports experiencing various symptoms of depression including dysphoric mood, a lack of drive, and negative self–thoughts. Debbie produced an elevated score on the new MMPI–A content scale Adolescent Alienation (A–aln). Adolescent girls who produce elevated scores on this scale report feeling emotionally distant from others, and they have low self–Esteem and poor social skills. Debbie's elevated score on the Adolescent Low Self–Esteem (A–lse) scale is consistent with numerous indications throughout her profile that she has a very low opinion of herself, that she tends to be overly self–critical, and that she is likely to be passive and submissive in interpersonal relationships.

Debbie's elevation on Adolescent School Problems (A–sch) indicates that she views the school environment very negatively and is likely to have poor academic accomplishments and disciplinary problems. Adolescents who produce elevated scores on this scale are prone to acting-out problems in school. However, in Debbie's case there are numerous indications in her MMPI–A profile that she does not engage in acting-out behaviors. Therefore, this descriptor would be inappropriate in this case. Debbie also produced an elevated score on Adolescent Low Aspiration (A–las). This indicates that she may presently have very low expectations for her future and that she is not very achievement–oriented at this time.

Debbie's MMPI–A profile is also noteworthy for a number of scales that are not elevated. Most notably, she produced a below average score on Adolescent Family Problems (A–fam). This indicates that Debbie reported experiencing fewer problems with members of her family and less familial strife and discord than did the average adolescent in the MMPI–A normative sample. This is clearly inconsistent with what is known about Debbie from her background and would suggest a tendency on her part to minimize family problems. It is likely that she is uncomfortable discussing her family background and difficulties and appears to have adopted a pattern whereby she externalizes her problems and attributes them to difficulties in school rather than in her home.

A positive indication in Debbie's MMPI–A profile is her relatively low score on Adolescent Negative Treatment Indicators (A–trt). Most adolescents who score as high as Debbie did on MMPI–A anxiety indicators tend to score considerably higher than she did on this scale. This indicates that, in spite of her social discomfort, Debbie may be willing to open up to a therapist. This issue will be discussed further under treatment recommendations.

Overall, Debbie's MMPI–A profile indicates that she is experiencing strong feelings of depression and anxiety at this time. Her mood is very dysphoric and she is experiencing some suicidal ideation. She likely feels fatigued and lacking in energy and is probably feeling very overwhelmed by her difficulties at this time. Debbie tends to be very uncomfortable around people and she likely avoids situations where there would be large crowds. She has a very negative self–view and tends to be very demanding of herself. However, because of her negative self–view Debbie expects to fail at what she attempts and is generally very pessimistic about her future. Debbie may also be inclined to engage in obsessive rumination about her difficulties. Debbie seems to view school as a major source of difficulty for her. On the other hand, she minimizes any problems she may have with members of her family. She tends to respond to psychological stress by developing physical symptoms or by becoming concerned about her physical health, and she likely has little insight into the connection between her psychological problems and physical symptoms.

Diagnostic Suggestions

Debbie's scores on the MMPI–A indicate a strong possibility that she is suffering from a mood disorder at this time. The possibility of a major depressive episode should be evaluated. Her scores also indicate that Debbie may be experiencing an anxiety disorder and that much of her anxiety seems to be focussed on school–related difficulties. The possibility of a social anxiety disorder should also be investigated. Debbie's pre–occupation with physical health concerns as well as her tendency to develop physical problems and concerns in response to stress suggest the possibility of a somatoform disorder. The possibility of an avoidant personality disorder needs also to be considered.

Treatment Recommendations

Specific treatment recommendations will obviously depend upon the final diagnosis and conceptualization in this case. Several issues need to be addressed in developing treatment recommendations. The possibility of a major depressive episode indicates that it would be desirable to refer Debbie for a psychiatric evaluation to determine whether medication is indicated. Individual therapy for Debbie's depression and deep–rooted social anxiety is also indicated. Debbie's failure to acknowledge her family problems indicates the need to work with her toward accepting these difficulties and understanding how they may be playing a role in her social anxiety and discomfort. Family therapy might also be explored in this case.

There are several indications in Debbie's MMPI–A profile that she is likely to benefit from therapy. First, Debbie's substantial psychological distress is likely to motivate her to seek and accept assistance in coping with her difficulties. Second, Debbie's relatively low score on A–trt indicates that she may be open to and receptive of therapeutic intervention at this time.

OUTCOME

Debbie was given the diagnoses of Specific Phobia, Situational Type–School and Major Depressive Disorder, Recurrent. Treatment interventions were coordinated with her pediatrician and school counselor. She was placed on antidepressant medication. In addition, she was seen in individual cognitive–behavioral therapy that incorporated desensitization techniques and assertiveness training to help Debbie deal with her social anxiety and discomfort. Debbie was also seen with her grandmother and mother in family therapy, and eventually she returned to school where she continued to have episodes of discomfort but was able first to tolerate and later to feel increasingly more comfortable in the school setting.

MMPI-A*

Extended Score Report

ID Number 4

Debbie

Female

Age 15

1/01/94

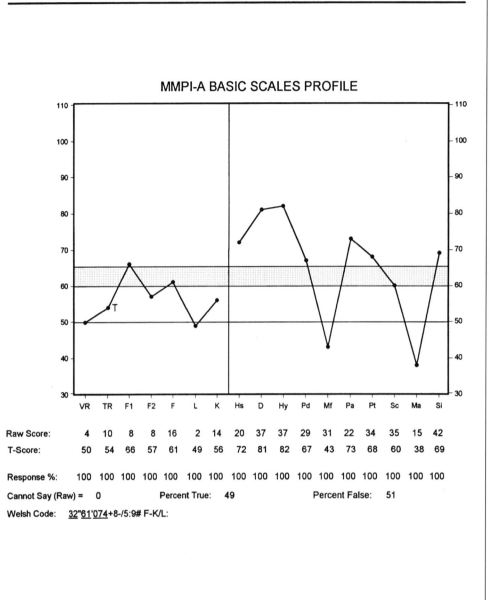

MMPI-A BASIC SCALES PROFILE

	VR	TR	F1	F2	F	L	K	Hs	D	Hy	Pd	Mf	Pa	Pt	Sc	Ma	Si
Raw Score:	4	10	8	8	16	2	14	20	37	37	29	31	22	34	35	15	42
T-Score:	50	54	66	57	61	49	56	72	81	82	67	43	73	68	60	38	69
Response %:	100	100	100	100	100	100	100	100	100	100	100	100	100	100	100	100	100

Cannot Say (Raw) = 0   Percent True: 49   Percent False: 51

Welsh Code: 32"61'074+8-/5:9# F-K/L:

CASE 4
"DEBBIE"

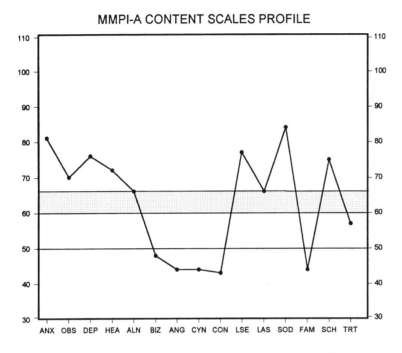

MMPI-A CONTENT SCALES PROFILE

	ANX	OBS	DEP	HEA	ALN	BIZ	ANG	CYN	CON	LSE	LAS	SOD	FAM	SCH	TRT
Raw Score:	19	13	21	21	11	3	7	10	5	14	10	20	9	13	13
T-Score:	81	70	76	72	66	48	44	44	43	77	66	84	44	75	57
Response %:	100	100	100	100	100	100	100	100	100	100	100	100	100	100	100

SUPPLEMENTARY SCORE REPORT

	Raw Score	T Score	Resp %
MacAndrew Alcoholism-Revised (MAC-R)	16	41	100
Alcohol/Drug Problem Acknowledgement (ACK)	2	43	100
Alcohol/Drug Problem Proneness (PRO)	16	48	100
Immaturity Scale (IMM)	17	58	100
Anxiety (A)	33	71	100
Repression (R)	19	66	100

Depression Subscales (Harris-Lingoes)

	Raw Score	T Score	Resp %
Subjective Depression (D1)	23	78	100
Psychomotor Retardation (D2)	10	78	100
Physical Malfunctioning (D3)	7	71	100
Mental Dullness (D4)	11	77	100
Brooding (D5)	8	70	100

Hysteria Subscales (Harris-Lingoes)

	Raw Score	T Score	Resp %
Denial of Social Anxiety (Hy1)	3	48	100
Need for Affection (Hy2)	5	50	100
Lassitude-Malaise (Hy3)	13	80	100
Somatic Complaints (Hy4)	12	73	100
Inhibition of Aggression (Hy5)	1	35	100

Psychopathic Deviate Subscales (Harris-Lingoes)

	Raw Score	T Score	Resp %
Familial Discord (Pd1)	5	56	100
Authority Problems (Pd2)	2	45	100
Social Imperturbability (Pd3)	2	43	100
Social Alienation (Pd4)	9	66	100
Self-Alienation (Pd5)	9	67	100

Paranoia Subscales (Harris-Lingoes)

	Raw Score	T Score	Resp %
Persecutory Ideas (Pa1)	6	57	100
Poignancy (Pa2)	7	67	100
Naivete (Pa3)	7	66	100

Schizophrenia Subscales (Harris-Lingoes)

Social Alienation (Sc1)	13	70	100
Emotional Alienation (Sc2)	7	76	100
Lack of Ego Mastery, Cognitive (Sc3)	5	58	100
Lack of Ego Mastery, Conative (Sc4)	12	78	100
Lack of Ego Mastery, Defective Inhibition (Sc5)	4	49	100
Bizarre Sensory Experiences (Sc6)	4	46	100

Hypomania Subscales (Harris-Lingoes)

Amorality (Ma1)	2	47	100
Psychomotor Acceleration (Ma2)	4	34	100
Imperturbability (Ma3)	3	50	100
Ego Inflation (Ma4)	2	35	100

Social Introversion Subscales (Ben-Porath, Hostetler, Butcher, & Graham)

Shyness / Self-Consciousness (Si1)	12	68	100
Social Avoidance (Si2)	6	72	100
Alienation--Self and Others (Si3)	10	55	100

Uniform T scores are used for Hs, D, Hy, Pd, Pa, Pt, Sc, Ma, and the Content Scales; all other
MMPI-A scales use linear T scores.

End of Report

SUGGESTED ITEMS FOR FOLLOW-UP

SUICIDAL BEHAVIORS

283. Most of the time I wish I were dead. (T)

SUICIDAL BEHAVIORS

CASE 5
"ERIC"

QUESTIONS REGARDING PSYCHOSIS IN A VIOLENCE-PRONE YOUNGSTER WITH POOR IMPULSE CONTROL

BACKGROUND

Eric, a 15-year-old, Caucasian boy, was admitted to a secure residential setting following homicidal threats made against his mother and younger sister. Before this admission, Eric was psychiatrically hospitalized seven times. The first hospitalization took place at age 11 following extremely aggressive behavior against his mother. His parents were divorced the following year. Each of the remaining hospitalizations has also been the result of assaultive or threatening behavior. Eric has destroyed furniture, thrown concrete blocks, set a room on fire, and threatened his mother and sister on two occasions, once with a knife and once with a rifle. He has a history of substance abuse which included inhalant abuse. He also has a history of having no friends as well as self-abusive behavior.

Eric was an unplanned child and his father had separated from his mother before his birth. The pregnancy and delivery were non-remarkable. Eric was diagnosed as having an irritable colon at age four months and chronic diarrhea until age four. Occasional enuretic episodes continued throughout his development. Eric's childhood behavior is described as being quite volatile, with frequent periods of becoming upset, even as a young child. Later, he would break windows and other objects in the house. Until the age of three, he would not sleep at night. He was described as having an extremely difficult temperament and was diagnosed as hyperactive at age three. Between the ages of three and five, he had extensive temper tantrums. At age five, he became involved in a serious physical altercation with peers. At age ten, Eric accused his father of sexual abuse but no charges were filed. At age eleven, he was seen by a child psychiatrist and given the diagnosis of Obsessive-Compulsive Disorder. In his first hospitalization, he was diagnosed as Bipolar Disorder and treated with Lithium with no significant results. Compliance with treatment has been extremely problematic.

There is a paternal history of mood disorder and substance abuse. In his last hospitalization, six months earlier, Eric was found to have a WISC-R verbal IQ of 108, a performance IQ of 102, and a full scale IQ of 105. His Bender Gestalt record was nonremarkable but did suggest impulsivity. The Rotter Incomplete Sentences Blank-High School Form indicated considerable anger. Projective drawings were quite primitive and suggested a thought disorder. The Rorschach, although a sparse record, was found to suggest a loss of reality testing, poorly modulated affect and a tendency to act out feelings.

Upon admission, Eric was observed to be of slight build and he appeared younger than his chronological age. His gait and posture were non-remarkable and there were no overt indications of gross or fine motor dysfunction. His speech was normal in tone, pacing, and volume. There were no indications of flight of ideas, loosening of associations, or tangentiality. His manner of interaction was quite guarded but his conversation became noticeably more animated when the topic turned to his thoughts of violence against others.

Eric presented a slightly flattened affect to a stated neutral mood. He denied experiencing, and there were no present indications of, hallucinations although he did vaguely relate one instance of hearing voices "outside" of his head during his last hospitalization. He attributed this experience to the medication that had been given to him. He was markedly paranoid, believing that "others" were conspiring against him. He indicated a belief that staff members of the facility were setting him up and that this was part of how people generally interacted with him. He stated that he believed that others were trying to control his thinking but denied a belief of thought insertion.

Eric expressed active homicidal ideation that was both specific to certain individuals and reflective of a generalized interest. He made specific threats to harm his sister and indicated a belief that killing her would be justified because "she makes my life miserable." When he was asked about potential methodologies of killing her, he listed various means that he had considered including beating her to death, poisoning her with household chemicals, and stabbing her with a kitchen knife. He stated that he did not care what would happen to him afterward and stated that "it didn't matter" because he could "always kill myself." Eric also made specific threats against a residential staff member whom he stated "has it in" for him. He detailed a plan of sneaking up

behind the person (who is hearing impaired) and hitting him over the head with a chair. He then related vivid imagery of the potential victim's broken skull and blood, and stated that this was enjoyable imagery. He also expressed a belief that killing was "fun" and that he fantasized about killing a series of people, "for fun."

Eric revealed a fascination with death and torture and related various thoughts of how to torture others. He then told how he had shot at birds with a slingshot and how he has set insects on fire. He also related enjoyment of self–asphyxiation and stated that he does this as often as he can. He denied autoerotic asphyxiation practices and denied sexual–sadistic fantasies. He denied active suicidal ideation or any history of suicidal behavior. He did not present with clinical indications of anxiety or phobias. He was clearly obsessed with violence but the obsession was not ego–dystonic to him. He was oriented to time, place, and person. His long-term, short-term, and immediate recall functions were clinically intact. His insight and judgment were markedly impaired.

MMPI–A INTERPRETATION
Profile Validity

Eric produced a valid MMPI–A profile. He responded to all but four of the test items and there was no consistent pattern among the items he omitted. However, in light of the referral issues it is noteworthy that Eric failed to respond to the items "I love my mother, or (if your mother is dead) I loved my mother" and "I have been disappointed in love."

Eric's scores on the MMPI–A consistency scales indicate that he was able to produce a coherent and consistent set of responses to the test items. He produced a moderately elevated score on F and his score on F_1 was considerably higher than his score on F_2. None of his elevations on these scales is sufficient to raise questions regarding the validity of his MMPI–A profile. However, it does appear that Eric responded more deviantly to items in the first part of the MMPI-A booklet. Overall, then, Eric's scores on the MMPI-A indicate that he cooperated with the testing procedure and that he reported experiencing some significant psychological problems.

Current Level of Adjustment

His MMPI-A profile indicates that although he likely exhibits very significant behavioral and emotional problems, Eric is not presently experiencing any anxiety or psychological distress. He produced little or no elevation on MMPI-A indicators of anxiety and relatively little elevation on the MMPI-A clinical scales. In contrast, Eric produced substantial elevation on the MMPI-A content scales, much of it indicating very substantial acting-out and impulse-control problems coupled with profound emotional alienation. Because of his serious impulse-control problems, Eric likely experiences significant behavioral problems. However, he does not appear to be concerned or anxious about the sequelae of these difficulties.

Symptoms and Traits

Eric's scores on the MMPI-A clinical scales indicate a pattern of chronic maladjustment. His elevation on Scales 4 and 8 indicates that Eric tends to be impulsive and to engage in significant acting-out behaviors, and that he likely has difficulties with individuals in positions of authority. Eric is prone to engage in fantasy and may experience psychotic symptomatology including delusional thinking. He is likely viewed by others as being isolated and aloof. His elevation on these scales indicates further that Eric is likely to have conflictual family relationships. He also tends to be self-centered and immature. Research indicates that some adolescent boys who produce this pattern of scores have been abused sexually in the past.

Eric's elevation on clinical Scale 6 and his pattern of scores on the relevant subscales indicate that he tends to be guarded, suspicious, and evasive and that he may experience paranoid delusional thinking.

Finally, Eric's elevation on Scale 2 indicates that he reports feeling some subjective depression at this time.

Eric's scores on the MMPI-A content scales provide a considerable amount of additional information about his psychological makeup and functioning. His most prominent elevation is on the Adolescent Alienation (A-aln) scale, an elevation indicating that Eric reports feeling considerable emotional distance from others. He believes that he cannot depend on others and that others cannot get close to or depend on him. He likely has substantial difficulties empathizing with others. Eric feels awkward in the presence of others and is likely to have few or no friends. Research indicates that adolescent boys who produce elevated scores on this scale are at risk for having substance-use problems.

Eric also produced a very elevated score on the Adolescent Low Aspirations (A-las) scale. This score indicates that Eric does not expect to succeed in life and has given up attempting to do so. He is likely to have minimal involvement in school activities, to have poor grades, and to experience disciplinary problems in school. Eric also produced an elevated score on the Adolescent Anger (A-ang) scale. His score on this scale indicates that Eric has substantial anger-control problems and that he is likely to have a history of assaultive, destructive acting-out behaviors. He is likely to throw tantrums when he perceives things as not going his way. Research indicates that, in clinical settings, boys who have elevated scores on this scale may have been abused sexually in the past. His elevated score on the Adolescent Conduct Problems (A-con) scale indicates that Eric is likely to display serious acting-out problems, that he may in the past or present have trouble with the law. He is likely to be disrespectful of others and he may enjoy causing others to be afraid of him "just for the fun of it."

Eric's elevated score on the Adolescent Family Problems (A-fam) scale indicates that he reports having serious difficulties with his parents and other members of his family, and that he likely perceives his family as lacking in love. He may report a considerable amount of familial discord. Examination of the list of Suggested Items for Follow–up indicates that one source of Eric's negative perception of his family life may be that he reports having gotten many beatings in the past. Eric's elevated score on Adolescent Social Discomfort (A–sod) indicates that he finds it difficult to be around others and that he tends to prefer to be by himself. Coupled with other indications in his profile, this elevation likely reflects Eric's inability to trust others or to form any meaningful emotional ties with people, including members of his own family.

Eric produced an elevated score on the Adolescent Bizarre Mentation (A–biz) scale. This score indicates that Eric reports having very strange thoughts and experiences that may include delusions and hallucinations. He may also harbor substantial paranoid delusional beliefs.

Eric's score on the supplementary MMPI–A Immaturity (IMM) scale indicates that he tends to be defiant and resistant, that he may enjoy teasing or bullying others, and that he is easily frustrated and quick to anger.

Overall, Eric's MMPI–A scores paint a very disturbing picture of this young man. He appears to have very serious impulse-control problems, a great deal of anger directed both inward and outward, and a tendency to disregard societal norms and standards and to act out against them. He feels alienated from members of his family as well as his peers, and does not appear to have a capacity or desire to form meaningful social relationships. He may derive pleasure from scaring or intimidating others. Eric appears to have given up hope of ever being able to develop social relationships, and he is generally pessimistic regarding his future. He views his family as a source of conflict and difficulty. Further, Eric experiences significant distortions in his reality testing and may harbor paranoid delusional beliefs regarding others in his environment. In spite of his current difficulties, Eric reports feeling little or no anxiety or distress.

Diagnostic Suggestions

Eric's MMPI–A profile suggests the possibility of a number of diagnoses. His possible psychotic symptoms and paranoid delusional thinking, coupled with substantial social and emotional alienation, suggest the need to consider seriously a diagnosis of schizophrenia or a related condition. Background information indicates that Eric may, in the past, have experienced a manic episode. Thus, the possibility of a schizoaffective disorder should also be considered. Eric's MMPI–A profile also shows very strong indications of a severe conduct disorder and the possibility of a schizoid or schizotypal personality disorder.

Eric's scores on the MMPI–A supplementary scales indicate the possibility of a substance-use disorder. His elevated scores on the Revised MacAndrew (MAC–R) and Alcohol/Drug Problem Proneness (PRO) scales indicate that Eric has personality and behavioral characteristics that place him at increased risk for developing an alcohol and/or drug problem. His score on the Alcohol/Drug Problem Acknowledgment (ACK) scale, indicates that Eric acknowledges only minor problems in this area. Examination of the list of Suggested Items for Follow–up indicates that Eric does report a number of potentially problematic tendencies and attitudes regarding alcohol and drugs.

Treatment Recommendations

Eric's MMPI–A profile indicates the need for an immediate psychiatric evaluation to determine whether anti–psychotic medication is indicated. Because of his severe distrust of others, Eric is not likely to do well in group therapy and the prospects for individual therapy also are limited. Setting up strict behavioral contingencies may be tried. However, Eric's lack of anxiety may limit the effectiveness of this intervention. It is unlikely that a therapist will be able to engage Eric in a meaningful therapeutic relationship, but an effort to do so would nevertheless be indicated. Should such a relationship develop, the possibility that Eric has been the victim of both physical and sexual abuse should be explored. It should be emphasized that Eric's MMPI–A scores, although suggestive of a history of physical and sexual abuse, can by no means be viewed as positive indications that abuse has occurred. Rather, they are best viewed as hypotheses in need of further examination. Finally, an elevated score on the Adolescent Negative Treatment Indicators (A–trt) scale, coupled with an absence of psychological distress or anxiety, indicate that Eric is not likely to be very motivated to pursue therapy at this time.

OUTCOME

Eric was given a diagnosis of Schizoaffective Disorder, Bipolar Type, with marked paranoid features and Conduct Disorder, Childhood Onset Type, Severe. He was assessed as being a significant risk of harm to others. He was seen as being in need of a highly structured behavioral therapy approach with clearly stated contingencies, gradually reduced limits occurring only when a combination of behavioral control, reduction of threats, compliance with treatment, and decrease in paranoia was manifested. Individual therapy using a cognitive–behavioral, anger-management approach together with expressive arts therapy was initiated. He was prescribed anti–psychotic, anti–manic, and anti–seizure medication, and he was referred for a substance-abuse evaluation as well as neuropsychological and neurological examinations. Eric was referred for family therapy and for a vocational evaluation.

Following his admission to the secure, residential treatment facility, Eric attacked another, smaller youth and bit him. He threatened to and attempted to attack a hearing-impaired staff member and continued to voice threats of killing his family and that staff member. He would spend much of his time drawing pictures of himself killing people. He refused any medication prescribed for him by his psychiatrist and refused neurological or neuropsychological examination. He refused all participation in therapy. He was discharged against the facility's advice by the custodial and placing agency.

MMPI-A*

Extended Score Report

ID Number 5

Eric

Male

Age 15

10/09/94

CASE 5
"ERIC"

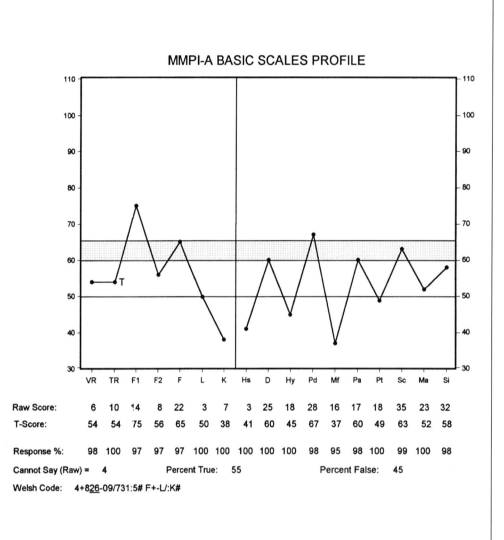

MMPI-A BASIC SCALES PROFILE

	VR	TR	F1	F2	F	L	K	Hs	D	Hy	Pd	Mf	Pa	Pt	Sc	Ma	Si
Raw Score:	6	10	14	8	22	3	7	3	25	18	28	16	17	18	35	23	32
T-Score:	54	54	75	56	65	50	38	41	60	45	67	37	60	49	63	52	58
Response %:	98	100	97	97	97	100	100	100	100	100	98	95	98	100	99	100	98

Cannot Say (Raw) = 4   Percent True: 55   Percent False: 45

Welsh Code: 4+8<u>26</u>-09/731:5# F+-L/:K#

CASE 5
"ERIC"

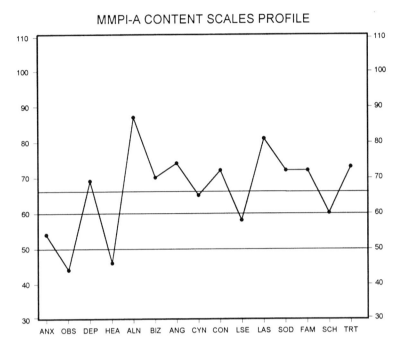

MMPI-A CONTENT SCALES PROFILE

	ANX	OBS	DEP	HEA	ALN	BIZ	ANG	CYN	CON	LSE	LAS	SOD	FAM	SCH	TRT
Raw Score:	10	5	16	5	16	10	14	18	17	8	12	17	22	10	17
T-Score:	54	44	69	46	87	70	74	65	72	58	81	72	72	60	73
Response %:	100	100	96	100	100	100	100	95	100	100	100	100	97	100	100

SUPPLEMENTARY SCORE REPORT

	Raw Score	T Score	Resp %
MacAndrew Alcoholism-Revised (MAC-R)	25	59	100
Alcohol/Drug Problem Acknowledgement (ACK)	6	59	100
Alcohol/Drug Problem Proneness (PRO)	21	60	100
Immaturity Scale (IMM)	26	70	100
Anxiety (A)	22	60	100
Repression (R)	10	42	100

Depression Subscales (Harris-Lingoes)

	Raw Score	T Score	Resp %
Subjective Depression (D1)	18	72	100
Psychomotor Retardation (D2)	6	56	100
Physical Malfunctioning (D3)	3	48	100
Mental Dullness (D4)	6	60	100
Brooding (D5)	6	66	100

Hysteria Subscales (Harris-Lingoes)

	Raw Score	T Score	Resp %
Denial of Social Anxiety (Hy1)	2	44	100
Need for Affection (Hy2)	5	50	100
Lassitude-Malaise (Hy3)	4	50	100
Somatic Complaints (Hy4)	4	50	100
Inhibition of Aggression (Hy5)	0	30	100

Psychopathic Deviate Subscales (Harris-Lingoes)

	Raw Score	T Score	Resp %
Familial Discord (Pd1)	6	64	100
Authority Problems (Pd2)	5	60	100
Social Imperturbability (Pd3)	1	35	100
Social Alienation (Pd4)	7	60	92
Self-Alienation (Pd5)	7	61	100

Paranoia Subscales (Harris-Lingoes)

	Raw Score	T Score	Resp %
Persecutory Ideas (Pa1)	11	75	100
Poignancy (Pa2)	4	55	100
Naivete (Pa3)	1	34	89

CASE 5
"ERIC"

Schizophrenia Subscales (Harris-Lingoes)
Social Alienation (Sc1)	14	74	95
Emotional Alienation (Sc2)	4	59	100
Lack of Ego Mastery, Cognitive (Sc3)	5	59	100
Lack of Ego Mastery, Conative (Sc4)	7	61	100
Lack of Ego Mastery, Defective Inhibition (Sc5)	3	48	100
Bizarre Sensory Experiences (Sc6)	3	44	100

Hypomania Subscales (Harris-Lingoes)
Amorality (Ma1)	5	66	100
Psychomotor Acceleration (Ma2)	5	43	100
Imperturbability (Ma3)	3	49	100
Ego Inflation (Ma4)	6	58	100

Social Introversion Subscales (Ben-Porath, Hostetler, Butcher, & Graham)
Shyness / Self-Consciousness (Si1)	8	56	100
Social Avoidance (Si2)	4	57	100
Alienation--Self and Others (Si3)	12	63	94

Uniform T scores are used for Hs, D, Hy, Pd, Pa, Pt, Sc, Ma, and the Content Scales; all other MMPI-A scales use linear T scores.

OMITTED ITEMS

The following items were omitted by the client. It may be helpful to discuss these item omissions with this individual to determine the reason for non-compliance with test instructions.

100. Most people are honest chiefly because they are afraid of being caught.
206. I have been disappointed in love.
230. I believe my sins are unpardonable.
258. I love my mother, or (if your mother is dead) I loved my mother.

End of Report

SUGGESTED ITEMS FOR FOLLOW-UP

ALCOHOL/DRUG PROBLEMS

247. I have used alcohol excessively. (T)

342. I can express my true feelings only when I drink. (T)

431. Talking over problems and worries with someone is often more helpful than taking drugs or medicines. (F)

FAMILY PROBLEMS

366. I have gotten many beatings. (T)

CASE 6
"FRANK"

A SEVERE CONDUCT DISORDER

BACKGROUND

Frank is a 16-year-old, Caucasian male referred for a psychological evaluation to ascertain treatment recommendations for extreme acting-out behaviors. He was recently placed in a psychiatric hospital by court order as part of a plea bargain that required that he undergo a thorough evaluation.

The referral records indicated that Frank had been adopted at age two and one-half. Nothing is known about his biological family. His adoptive parents divorced when he was six years old. His foster parents described his early childhood behavior as being primarily unsocialized. During his primary school years, he was diagnosed as having a learning disability and was placed in Learning Disabled programming but was mainstreamed during middle school. It was at this time that his behavioral problems became evident. During high school, his acting–out behavior was described as being extreme. He has made inappropriate sexual comments to girls and female teachers and frequently provokes his peers into fighting with him.

An incident was described in which Frank set a girl's hair afire in class. He has frequently been involved in theft. It is also indicated that he has killed a cat with an ax

and attacked a peer with a burning ember from a campfire when the peer tried to intervene to save the animal. He has had three previous psychiatric hospitalizations and numerous group-home placements. He has carried the diagnosis of Attention Deficit Disorder with Hyperactivity and Conduct Disorder.

Frank appeared to be his stated age. His clothing was clean, somewhat disheveled, and appropriate to the season. His hygiene and grooming were adequate. His gait and posture were non-remarkable, and there were no overt indications of gross or fine motor dysfunction. His speech was normal in tone, pacing, and volume. His verbalizations were coherent, goal–directed, and made use of abstractions. There were no indications of loosening of associations, flight of ideas, or tangentiality. His eye contact was direct and his attention span was adequate. He described himself frequently as being "patient smart" and indicated that he "knew all the right things to say" to mental-health clinicians.

Frank presented an appropriate affect to a stated neutral mood. He denied experiencing, and there were no current indications of, hallucinations, delusions or organized paranoid ideation. He did report periods of some depression and that he has cut himself when he gets moody and angry. However, he denied any history of actual suicidal behavior and denied present suicidal ideation. He denied disturbances in his sleep, health, or appetite. Frank denied current thoughts of wanting to harm anyone but did state that he sees himself as having a problem with anger. He stated that his anger will, at times, become focussed on a particular individual, and that is when he will act out. Frank claimed that he will, at such times, lose control of his emotions. However, his descriptions of such behavior gave the appearance of being generally goal directed and instrumental.

Frank reported a history of fire-setting, making bombs, and using fire for revenge when angry. He disclaimed any compulsive urge to set fires or fascination with fire, but admitted to an interest in fire. There were no indications of phobias, obsessions, or compulsions. He was oriented to time, place, and person. His immediate, long-term and short-term recall functions were intact. He was able to interpret proverbs and identify similarities between related objects. His insight and judgment appeared to be quite limited.

Frank was administered a battery of psychological tests consisting of the Rorschach Inkblot Technique, the Bender Visual Motor Gestalt Test, the Thematic Apperception Test, Projective Drawings, and the MMPI–A. Using the Koppitz scoring system, Frank's Bender record was found to indicate an age-appropriate level of visual motor perceptual developmental functioning. Qualitatively, the record suggested impulsivity. The Projective Drawings suggested a fairly barren interpersonal view and a likelihood of depression and anxiety. Socially, he is likely to be quite egocentric. Projective personality assessment found that Frank's record was similar to youth who evidence emotional dyscontrol and acting out of conflicts. No indications of a psychosis were suggested by the record, but there were indications of underlying depression and anxiety.

Interpersonally, Frank is likely to be seen as oppositional and defiant.

MMPI–A INTERPRETATION
Profile Validity

Frank produced a valid MMPI–A profile. He responded to all the test items and provided a consistent and coherent set of responses. There are no indications of any deviant response patterns. Frank's cooperative approach to the testing can be viewed as a positive indication of his overall approach to this evaluation.

Current Level of Adjustment

Frank's MMPI–A profile indicates that he is not experiencing considerable psychological distress at this time. He produced only one prominently elevated clinical scale with two secondary elevations and a similar pattern on the content scales. His scores on clinical Scales 2 and 7 are both within normal limits, indicating that Frank does not report many symptoms of anxiety or distress at this time. Frank's problems appear to be relatively focussed and circumscribed and are likely to be manifested primarily in externalizing behavior.

Symptoms and Traits

Frank's prominent elevation on the MMPI–A clinical Scale 4 indicates that he is prone to acting-out and delinquent behavior. He likely resents authority, has academic problems in school, and has considerable conflict with his family. Frank's elevation on this scale indicates further that he may have alcohol or drug problems and that he tends to be impulsive and aggressive. Frank is also not likely to accept responsibility for his own behavior. Examination of Frank's scores on the subscales for Scale 4 supports the interpretation that he tends to have conflicts with authority figures and with members of his family. These scores also indicate that Frank likely presents himself in a socially poised manner and that he may create an initially favorable impression upon others.

Frank produced a secondary elevation on clinical Scale 9. This provides further support for the indication that Frank is prone to impulsive, acting-out behavior and that he is at risk for a substance-use problem. He likely presents with an unrealistically positive self–view that may mask insecurities. Frank also produced a very low score on Scale 0, indicating that he feels very comfortable in social situations and is likely viewed by others initially as friendly and outgoing.

Frank's scores on the MMPI–A content scales provide further information regarding his current psychological functioning. His most prominent elevation was on the Adolescent Family Problems (A–fam) scale. This indicates that Frank perceives his family very negatively, as a source of conflict and strife, and that he likely gets into frequent arguments and disputes with members of his family. Frank's highly elevated score on this scale indicates further that he views his family as lacking in love, and that he does not believe that he can turn to family members for support or comfort. He believes that he has frequently been punished without cause, and that he is treated more like a child than an adult. Examination of the list of Suggested Items for Follow–up indicates that Frank reports that he has frequently been beaten, presumably by one or both of his parents.

Frank also produced an elevated score on the Adolescent Cynicism (A–cyn) scale. This score indicates that Frank is very untrusting of the motives of other people, and that he views the world as hostile and unsupporting. Frank's elevation on this scale indicates further that he believes that others will use unfair means to get ahead in life and that others tend to be jealous of him and his accomplishments. Frank's elevated score on the Adolescent School Problems (A–sch) scale, indicates that he reports experiencing a variety of problems in school, that he likely has poor academic accomplishments, and that he tends to pose a significant disciplinary problem to teachers and school administrators.

Finally, Frank produced a moderately elevated score on the Adolescent Conduct Problems (A–con) scale, indicating that, although he acknowledges having some acting-out problems, the number and severity of problems that he reports are inconsistent with objective indications of the severity of his acting-out tendencies. Thus, Frank appears to minimize the severity of his behavioral problems.

Overall, Frank's MMPI–A scales indicate that he is prone to considerable acting-out problems, that he is impulsive and irresponsible, and that Frank tends to minimize the severity of his behavioral acting-out problems. Frank is resentful of, and tends to get in conflicts with, authority figures, and he is very unhappy with his relationship with his family. He likely perceives his home environment as hostile and non–supportive, and he believes that he has frequently been mistreated by members of his family. Outwardly, Frank is likely to appear very friendly, socially poised, and outgoing, and he may make a favorable first impression. However, Frank has a very negative view of people and their motives, and it is very difficult for him to form close relationships or for others to get close to him.

Diagnostic Suggestions

The primary diagnostic indication in Frank's MMPI–A profile is a conduct disorder. There are no indications of a mood or anxiety disorder and no signs of any deficits in reality testing.

Along with the possibility of a conduct disorder, Frank's MMPI–A profile indicates that he is at substantial risk for developing a substance-use problem. His score on the Revised MacAndrew (MAC–R) scale indicates that Frank possesses numerous personality characteristics, most notably a tendency toward risk–taking and sensation-seeking, that place him at considerable risk for developing a substance-use problem. Frank also produced an elevated score on the new Alcohol/Drug Problem Proneness (PRO) scale. This scale, like MAC–R, indicates the presence of personality characteristics and behavioral tendencies that place an adolescent at significant risk for developing a substance-use problem. An elevated score on PRO indicates that Frank may tend to become involved with negative peer groups that may engage in alcohol or drug abuse.

It should be emphasized that elevated scores on these two scales, in themselves, are not sufficient to indicate that Frank actually does have alcohol or drug problems. However, they do indicate that he is at substantial risk for developing such problems and this possibility should be examined further.

Although Frank produced elevated scores on both MMPI–A substance-use risk indicators, he does not acknowledge having substantial problems in this area. His score on the Alcohol/Drug Problem Acknowledgment (ACK) scale falls well within normal limits. Frank's lack of elevation on this scale does not mean that he does not have problems in this area. Rather, this score tells us only that Frank does not acknowledge difficulties in this area. If objective, non–test data were to indicate that Frank does indeed have an alcohol- or drug-use problem, then his score on ACK can be viewed as an indication that Frank minimizes or denies his difficulties in this area.

Treatment Suggestions

The primary focus of any treatment plan is likely to be Frank's acting-out tendencies and behaviors. His very high score on A–fam suggests the possibility that family difficulties lie at the core of his acting-out behavior, and that, over the long term, family therapy may be the most efficacious treatment modality.

More immediately, setting up a contingency–based behavior management program may help reduce the likelihood that Frank will engage in extreme acting-out behavior. However, it would be very important that such a program be negotiated with Frank, and that he not perceive it as yet another attempt by authority figures to control his behavior. Moreover, developing a relationship with a caring individual therapist may help disabuse Frank of some of his cynical, misanthropic views and beliefs about people.

His relatively low score on the Adolescent Negative Treatment Indicators (A–trt) scale, coupled with his overall cooperative approach to this evaluation, indicate that Frank may, at this time, be open to therapeutic intervention.

OUTCOME

Frank received a diagnosis of Conduct Disorder, Childhood Onset Type. No conclusive information was obtained to indicate whether Frank had a substance-use problem. He was placed first in a closed residential setting on a program with specific contingencies. He was also seen in individual therapy with a focus upon anger management and thinking errors. Despite significant problems at the outset of therapy, Frank eventually developed a positive relationship with his therapist. He was subsequently transferred to an open setting where he excelled in the vocational programming. He was later successfully mainstreamed into public schools and eventually transferred to a group home where he also did quite well. Recommended family therapy was not pursued because of an unwillingness on the part of Frank's adoptive family members to participate.

MMPI-A*

Extended Score Report

ID Number 6

Frank

Male

Age 16

4/02/93

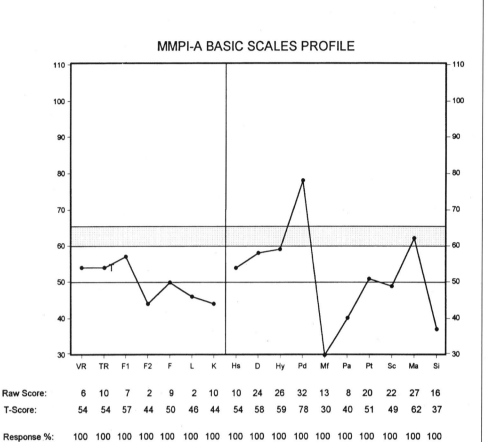

MMPI-A BASIC SCALES PROFILE

	VR	TR	F1	F2	F	L	K	Hs	D	Hy	Pd	Mf	Pa	Pt	Sc	Ma	Si
Raw Score:	6	10	7	2	9	2	10	10	24	26	32	13	8	20	22	27	16
T-Score:	54	54	57	44	50	46	44	54	58	59	78	30	40	51	49	62	37
Response %:	100	100	100	100	100	100	100	100	100	100	100	100	100	100	100	100	100

Cannot Say (Raw) =   0   Percent True: 51   Percent False: 49

Welsh Code: 4'+9-3217/86:05# F/LK:

CASE 6
"FRANK"

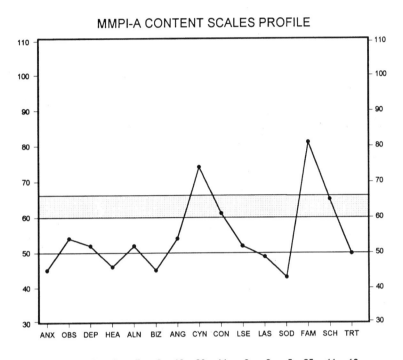

MMPI-A CONTENT SCALES PROFILE

	ANX	OBS	DEP	HEA	ALN	BIZ	ANG	CYN	CON	LSE	LAS	SOD	FAM	SCH	TRT
Raw Score:	6	9	9	5	7	2	10	20	14	6	6	5	25	11	10
T-Score:	45	54	52	46	52	45	54	74	61	52	49	43	81	65	50
Response %:	100	100	100	100	100	100	100	100	100	100	100	100	100	100	100

SUPPLEMENTARY SCORE REPORT

	Raw Score	T Score	Resp %
MacAndrew Alcoholism-Revised (MAC-R)	30	70	100
Alcohol/Drug Problem Acknowledgement (ACK)	5	54	100
Alcohol/Drug Problem Proneness (PRO)	24	67	100
Immaturity Scale (IMM)	17	56	100
Anxiety (A)	13	48	100
Repression (R)	12	47	100

Depression Subscales (Harris-Lingoes)

	Raw Score	T Score	Resp %
Subjective Depression (D1)	10	53	100
Psychomotor Retardation (D2)	6	56	100
Physical Malfunctioning (D3)	4	55	100
Mental Dullness (D4)	6	60	100
Brooding (D5)	2	46	100

Hysteria Subscales (Harris-Lingoes)

	Raw Score	T Score	Resp %
Denial of Social Anxiety (Hy1)	6	66	100
Need for Affection (Hy2)	4	46	100
Lassitude-Malaise (Hy3)	8	66	100
Somatic Complaints (Hy4)	4	50	100
Inhibition of Aggression (Hy5)	2	44	100

Psychopathic Deviate Subscales (Harris-Lingoes)

	Raw Score	T Score	Resp %
Familial Discord (Pd1)	7	69	100
Authority Problems (Pd2)	7	73	100
Social Imperturbability (Pd3)	6	67	100
Social Alienation (Pd4)	4	46	100
Self-Alienation (Pd5)	7	61	100

Paranoia Subscales (Harris-Lingoes)

	Raw Score	T Score	Resp %
Persecutory Ideas (Pa1)	3	46	100
Poignancy (Pa2)	3	49	100
Naivete (Pa3)	1	34	100

CASE 6
"FRANK"

Schizophrenia Subscales (Harris-Lingoes)

Social Alienation (Sc1)	7	53	100
Emotional Alienation (Sc2)	3	54	100
Lack of Ego Mastery, Cognitive (Sc3)	4	55	100
Lack of Ego Mastery, Conative (Sc4)	6	57	100
Lack of Ego Mastery, Defective Inhibition (Sc5)	1	38	100
Bizarre Sensory Experiences (Sc6)	3	44	100

Hypomania Subscales (Harris-Lingoes)

Amorality (Ma1)	3	52	100
Psychomotor Acceleration (Ma2)	8	57	100
Imperturbability (Ma3)	5	62	100
Ego Inflation (Ma4)	7	64	100

Social Introversion Subscales (Ben-Porath, Hostetler, Butcher, & Graham)

Shyness / Self-Consciousness (Si1)	1	33	100
Social Avoidance (Si2)	1	43	100
Alienation--Self and Others (Si3)	8	51	100

Uniform T scores are used for Hs, D, Hy, Pd, Pa, Pt, Sc, Ma, and the Content Scales; all other
MMPI-A scales use linear T scores.

End of Report

SUGGESTED ITEMS FOR FOLLOW-UP

ALCOHOL/DRUG PROBLEMS

247. I have used alcohol excessively. (T)

FAMILY PROBLEMS

366. I have gotten many beatings. (T)

440. I have spent nights away from home when my parents did not know where I was. (T)

CASE 7
"GREG"

A CASE OF COMPULSIVE MASTURBATION

BACKGROUND

Greg is a 15-year-old, Caucasian male who was admitted to residential treatment by court order. Presenting problems included sexually offending against his younger sister, physical aggression, and school behavioral problems.

Greg's parents are both mildly mentally retarded. In addition, his mother has a severe speech impediment. His sister, who is three years younger than Greg, is also mildly mentally retarded. Greg is reported to have been born after a normal pregnancy and delivery. He apparently achieved developmental milestones normally. He was diagnosed as being hyperactive while in the third grade. It was also during this time that he was reportedly sexually abused by his uncle. Previous intelligence testing using the WISC-R found Greg to have a verbal IQ of 82, a performance IQ of 85, and a full scale IQ of 82.

Upon placement in the residential center, Greg was initially compliant with his treatment. However, he quickly alienated himself from his peers by openly masturbating. Although that behavior was eliminated, he continued to be ridiculed and rejected by his peers. He also frequently sought attention and would talk incessantly to anyone.

His limited social skills resulted in Greg being ostracized even more. He frequently would explode with considerable rage and destroyed furniture on occasion. In another instance, Greg made a false allegation of rape against three peers who had attacked him. It was also ascertained that on home visits, which were subsequently discontinued, Greg would drink beer and watch X–rated movies with his father.

Midway through treatment, Greg came to the nurse's office and complained of a swollen scrotum and pain. He was seen by the physician with a diagnosis of epididymis. He was admitted to the hospital for emergency surgery where a scrotal exploration found right testicle torsion, secondary to masturbation, and a right orchidectomy was performed. Following his discharge back to the residential facility, Greg was referred for a comprehensive psychological evaluation.

During his clinical interview, Greg was observed to be dressed in street clothing which was somewhat dirty and disheveled. His hygiene and grooming were adequate. His gait and posture were non-remarkable. His speech was somewhat rapid, variable in tone, and normal in volume. His verbalizations were highly concrete and mildly tangential. There were no indications of loosening of associations or flight of ideas. His manner of social interaction was polite and cooperative, but he was observed to be considerably guarded concerning his sexual ideation. He did affirm continued fantasies and indicated that he still masturbates three to five times per day. He indicated that he masturbates when he feels anxious as well as when he feels sexually stimulated. He indicated that sexual stimulation for him included both nonviolent and violent sexual fantasies. He also reported periodic nightmares involving himself and various horror movie genre characters. He denied any masturbatory fantasies concerning young children.

Greg was administered a battery of psychological tests consisting of the Rorschach Inkblot Technique, the Bender Visual Motor Gestalt Test, the House Tree Person, the Thematic Apperception Test, Kinetic Family Drawings, and the MMPI–A. Projective assessment found that Greg tends to see the world in a manner that is different from others and that he may be prone to regression into fantasy. Such regression may be suggestive of episodic poor ties with reality and may be especially keyed by emotionally laden stressors. His manner of thinking is suggested to be extremely concrete with poor attention to detail. His coping skills appear to be quite limited. He appears to be an individual with limited animation in thought and behavior and who tends to evidence stereotypic thinking. The record suggests considerable anxiety with a predominant emotional theme of depression. Greg evidences poor emotional integration with a tendency to attempt to over-control his hostile impulses. He presents with extreme dependency needs and the record is further suggestive of considerable conflict over sexual activity. Interpersonally, Greg appears to feel inadequate and insecure. He sees women as more powerful than he. He appears to be quite mistrusting of others.

MMPI–A INTERPRETATION
Profile Validity

Greg produced a valid MMPI–A profile. However, his pattern of scores on the validity scales indicates that he approached the test in a guarded and defensive manner. Such an approach is relatively uncommon for adolescents, particularly in clinical settings.

Greg responded to all the MMPI–A test items, and his scores on the consistency scales indicate that he was able to produce a consistent and coherent set of responses. His scores on F and its subscales indicate that Greg did not report experiencing many psychological problems. He produced moderately elevated scores on both L and K. Whenever a deviant pattern of scores on these scales is observed in an MMPI–A profile, it is particularly important to examine the adolescent's score on TRIN to determine whether a response set may have contributed to scores on L and K. This is because all of the items on L and all but one of the items on K are keyed "false." In this case, Greg's T score on TRIN is 51, and we can rule out a response set as a contributing factor to Greg's elevations on L and K.

Another possible cause for moderately elevated scores on L is growing up in a very traditional home. Adolescents who come from such homes tend to score somewhat higher than average on L because they endorse some of the L items that are consistent with their moral or religious upbringing. In this case, background information indicates that Greg was not raised in a very traditional home and this interpretation is ruled out.

Thus, Greg's elevations on L and K are most reasonably interpreted as indicating that he approached the test in a guarded and defensive manner, that Greg attempted to portray himself in an overly positive way by denying minor faults and shortcomings that most adolescents will readily acknowledge, and that Greg likely has limited insight into his psychological problems.

Current Level of Adjustment

In spite of his defensive approach to the test, Greg produced considerable elevation on a number of the clinical scales and secondary elevations on others. He produced considerably fewer elevations on the content scales. Among the clinical scales, Greg's elevated scales included 2 and 7, indicating that he acknowledges experiencing some psychological distress at this time. His pattern of scores on the clinical scales is characterized by a negative slope, with most of his elevations on the left-hand side of the clinical scale profile. This is suggestive of a "neurotic" condition in which Greg may have substantial psychological problems, primarily of an internalizing nature. However, his reality testing is likely to be generally intact. His elevated score on Scale 4 indicates that in addition to emotional difficulties, Greg likely engages in substantial acting out. Thus, Greg's scores are indicative of both internalizing and externalizing problems.

Symptoms and Traits

Greg produced primary elevations on clinical scales 1, 2, 3, and 4. In interpreting his elevation on these scales, particularly 1 and 3, Greg's recent medical problems need to be considered. We know from the background information that Greg has recently undergone surgery in which a right orchidectomy was performed. This could account for some elevation on scales related to physical health problems and concerns. However, Greg's elevations on Scales 1 and 3 exceed considerably what would be expected on the basis of his recent surgery.

Thus, beyond the obvious physical problems related to his recent surgery, Greg appears to be preoccupied with physical health concerns, and he is likely to complain about a variety of somatic problems that tend to be somewhat vague in nature. His elevation on Scale 1 indicates further that it is likely that Greg is seen by others as self-centered and demanding, and that he is likely to have school problems including academic and disciplinary difficulties.

Examination of Greg's scores on the subscales of Scale 2 indicates that a considerable proportion of his elevation on this scale is likely attributable to physical health concerns and complaints. However, Greg also reports experiencing symptoms of depression, including dysphoric mood and feelings of hopelessness and dissatisfaction. Greg likely displays a general apathy and lack of interest in activities. It is likely he is lacking in self-confidence and is socially awkward and withdrawn.

As noted, Greg's elevation on Scale 3 reflects an excessive preoccupation with somatic concerns. It also suggests that Greg is prone to developing physical health problems or concerns in response to stress. His elevation on this scale suggests further that Greg has a strong need for attention and approval, that he is likely to be viewed by others as immature, and that he likely has limited insight into his problem areas.

Greg's elevated score on Scale 4 indicates that he is likely to display acting-out, aggressive behaviors. Greg is likely to have difficulties incorporating the values of society, and he is likely to be rebellious toward figures of authority. He likely shows very poor impulse control, poor planning ability, and a low tolerance for boredom and frustration. Greg's score on this scale indicates further that he may have significant family conflict and that he may be at risk for developing a substance-use problem. Research indicates that adolescents tested in clinical settings who produce elevated scores on Scale 4 may have a history of having been sexually abused. Finally, Greg's elevated score on Scale 4 is consistent with other MMPI–A indicators suggesting that he tends to be egocentric and selfish.

Greg's secondary elevation on Scale 7 indicates that he is experiencing some tension and anxiety at this time. However, his scores on the other elevated clinical scales suggest that Greg responds to these experiences by focussing on physical health concerns and that he may have difficulty recognizing the psychological component of these emotions. This interpretation is supported by the absence of elevation in Greg's scores on the Welsh Anxiety scale and the Adolescent Anxiety (A-anx) content scale, both of which focus more on subjective feelings of anxiety. Finally, his elevated score on Scale 0 supports indications in some of the more prominently elevated clinical scales that Greg is awkward and uncomfortable in social situations and that he is insecure and lacking in self-confidence.

Greg's pattern of scores on the MMPI-A content scales provides further insight into his current functioning, particularly as seen from his perspective. As discussed in the introduction, because of their greater homogeneity and the very obvious quality of their items, the MMPI-A content scales provide a more direct means of communication between the test-taker and interpreter than do the more heterogeneous clinical scales. In protocols such as Greg's, that are characterized by a defensive approach, this usually means that there will be relatively little interpretive material in the content scales. However, Greg did produce some elevations on a few content scales, offering us an opportunity to view his problems from his perspective.

Greg's most prominent elevation is on the Adolescent Health Concerns (A-hea) scale. As was the case with his elevations on clinical scales 1 and 3, his level of elevation on A-hea exceeds what would be expected based on his actual recent physical health problems. Thus, Greg's content scales confirm that he tends to focus his attention on physical health problems and tends to deny or minimize psychological difficulties. Further, he is likely to reject psychological interpretations of his problems.

Greg also produced an elevated score on the Adolescent Low Aspirations (A-las) scale. This score indicates that Greg is rather pessimistic about his prospects for the future and that he likely is disinterested in school activities and shows poor academic performance. Greg's moderate elevation on the Adolescent Depression (A-dep) scale indicates that he acknowledges experiencing some dysphoria at this time.

Greg's moderate elevation on the Adolescent Family Problems scale (A-fam) reflects his acknowledgment that there is currently some conflict and turmoil in his family. He may feel somewhat alienated from members of his family and does not believe that he can turn to them for support. This pattern is certainly consistent with background information indicating that the immediate precipitator of Greg's hospitalization was his sexually abusing his younger, mildly mentally retarded sister. In fact, in light of this information, a greater degree of elevation on A-fam would be expected. Thus, Greg's moderate elevation on this scale, coupled with background information, suggests that although he acknowledges some difficulties in this area, he tends to minimize problems that he is experiencing with members of his family.

Finally, Greg's elevated score on the supplementary MMPI-A Welsh Repression scale is consistent with other indicators in his profile suggesting that Greg tends to be emotionally overcontrolled, that he shows few if any emotions, and that he has a generally pessimistic and defeatist attitude.

In sum, Greg's MMPI-A profile indicates that he is very focussed on somatic complaints and concerns, that he tends to respond to stress by developing physical symptoms or complaints, that he is psychologically very immature and naive, that he lacks insight into his problems and that he tends to reject psychological explanations of his difficulties. It is likely that Greg is viewed by others as self-centered and selfish, and he is very needy and demanding of attention. He may have a very low tolerance for frustration and is likely to act out impulsively in response to seemingly minor provocation. Greg tends to be very pessimistic and insecure, and he may acknowledge some symptoms of depression at this time. However, in general, he is likely to have great difficulties identifying and understanding his emotions, and he is inclined to minimize or deny psychological difficulties. He feels socially awkward, and because of his aggressive acting-out tendencies he is likely to have difficulties forming and maintaining social ties.

Diagnostic Suggestions

Greg's MMPI–A profile suggests a number of possible diagnoses for further exploration. His negatively sloped clinical scale profile suggests a neurotic disorder. Greg does acknowledge some depressive symptoms at this time, and he tends to hold a very negative, self–depreciatory self–view. It is possible that both his somatic preoccupation and acting-out tendencies may be related to an underlying long–standing depressive disorder. Greg's elevation on Scale 4 also indicates the likelihood of a conduct disorder. His tendency to focus on somatic problems and complaints suggests the possibility of a somatoform disorder.

Treatment Recommendations

Greg's MMPI–A profile indicates a number of recommendations to be considered in devising a treatment plan for him. His combination of externalizing and internalizing problems suggests that a combined treatment approach may be indicated. Behavioral management techniques may be used to deal with the more immediate acting-out problems whereas a more long–term approach, focussed on helping Greg recognize, accept, and respond appropriately to his emotions, may help address some of the core issues that may underlie his acting-out behaviors. Social-skills training may help Greg overcome some of his social awkwardness and discomfort. In developing his treatment plan, Greg's reluctance to accept psychological interpretations of his problems, and his concomitant lack of insight, should be brought to the attention of the therapist.

OUTCOME

Greg received a diagnosis of Attention Deficit Hyperactivity Disorder, NOS; Conduct Disorder, Adolescent Onset Type; and Dysthymia. He was referred to a specialized behavioral sexual offender treatment program on an outpatient basis while he received individual therapy at the residential facility. Treatment focussed on social-skill development and anger management. Greg was eventually discharged to a group home with a recommendation that he continue to receive individual therapy for his dysthymic disorder.

MMPI-A*

Extended Score Report

ID Number 7

Greg

Male

Age 15

4/15/93

CASE 7
"GREG"

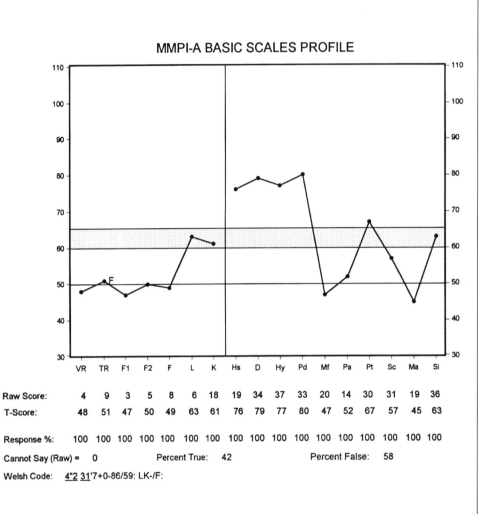

MMPI-A BASIC SCALES PROFILE

	VR	TR	F1	F2	F	L	K	Hs	D	Hy	Pd	Mf	Pa	Pt	Sc	Ma	Si
Raw Score:	4	9	3	5	8	6	18	19	34	37	33	20	14	30	31	19	36
T-Score:	48	51	47	50	49	63	61	76	79	77	80	47	52	67	57	45	63
Response %:	100	100	100	100	100	100	100	100	100	100	100	100	100	100	100	100	100

Cannot Say (Raw) =   0   Percent True: 42   Percent False: 58

Welsh Code: 4"2 31'7+0-86/59: LK-/F:

CASE 7
"GREG"

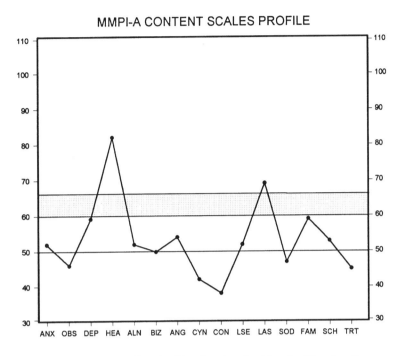

MMPI-A CONTENT SCALES PROFILE

	ANX	OBS	DEP	HEA	ALN	BIZ	ANG	CYN	CON	LSE	LAS	SOD	FAM	SCH	TRT
Raw Score:	9	6	12	23	7	4	10	9	4	6	10	7	17	8	7
T-Score:	52	46	59	82	52	50	54	42	38	52	69	47	59	53	45
Response %:	100	100	100	100	100	100	100	100	100	100	100	100	100	100	100

SUPPLEMENTARY SCORE REPORT

	Raw Score	T Score	Resp %
MacAndrew Alcoholism-Revised (MAC-R)	25	59	100
Alcohol/Drug Problem Acknowledgement (ACK)	2	42	100
Alcohol/Drug Problem Proneness (PRO)	17	51	100
Immaturity Scale (IMM)	11	46	100
Anxiety (A)	14	49	100
Repression (R)	20	65	100

Depression Subscales (Harris-Lingoes)

	Raw Score	T Score	Resp %
Subjective Depression (D1)	17	70	100
Psychomotor Retardation (D2)	9	71	100
Physical Malfunctioning (D3)	7	75	100
Mental Dullness (D4)	7	64	100
Brooding (D5)	5	61	100

Hysteria Subscales (Harris-Lingoes)

	Raw Score	T Score	Resp %
Denial of Social Anxiety (Hy1)	4	55	100
Need for Affection (Hy2)	8	63	100
Lassitude-Malaise (Hy3)	11	77	100
Somatic Complaints (Hy4)	8	64	100
Inhibition of Aggression (Hy5)	3	51	100

Psychopathic Deviate Subscales (Harris-Lingoes)

	Raw Score	T Score	Resp %
Familial Discord (Pd1)	5	59	100
Authority Problems (Pd2)	6	67	100
Social Imperturbability (Pd3)	3	48	100
Social Alienation (Pd4)	8	65	100
Self-Alienation (Pd5)	9	69	100

Paranoia Subscales (Harris-Lingoes)

	Raw Score	T Score	Resp %
Persecutory Ideas (Pa1)	5	53	100
Poignancy (Pa2)	2	42	100
Naivete (Pa3)	4	50	100

**CASE 7
"GREG"**

Schizophrenia Subscales (Harris-Lingoes)

Social Alienation (Sc1)	11	65	100
Emotional Alienation (Sc2)	3	54	100
Lack of Ego Mastery, Cognitive (Sc3)	3	50	100
Lack of Ego Mastery, Conative (Sc4)	7	61	100
Lack of Ego Mastery, Defective Inhibition (Sc5)	4	53	100
Bizarre Sensory Experiences (Sc6)	4	47	100

Hypomania Subscales (Harris-Lingoes)

Amorality (Ma1)	2	45	100
Psychomotor Acceleration (Ma2)	6	48	100
Imperturbability (Ma3)	4	55	100
Ego Inflation (Ma4)	2	37	100

Social Introversion Subscales (Ben-Porath, Hostetler, Butcher, & Graham)

Shyness / Self-Consciousness (Si1)	7	53	100
Social Avoidance (Si2)	1	43	100
Alienation--Self and Others (Si3)	10	57	100

Uniform T scores are used for Hs, D, Hy, Pd, Pa, Pt, Sc, Ma, and the Content Scales; all other MMPI-A scales use linear T scores.

End of Report

SUGGESTED ITEMS FOR FOLLOW-UP

FAMILY PROBLEMS

366. I have gotten many beatings. (T)

460. I have never run away from home. (F)

CASE 8
"HENRY"

COURT-ORDERED EVALUATION OF
AN ASSAULTIVE YOUNGSTER

BACKGROUND

Henry is a 14-year-old, African American male referred by a juvenile court judge for a pre-sentence investigation evaluation having been found guilty of aggravated assault. Henry had seriously injured an adolescent boy whom he believed had stolen his jacket. Because he had a history of psychological problems and treatment, the judge requested a pre-sentence psychological evaluation to assist her in determining whether Henry should be incarcerated or committed for residential treatment.

Henry has had two previous psychiatric hospitalizations, the last following a suicide attempt by hanging in a closet. The social history indicated a record of disruptive behavior, chronic maladjustment, and a series of four deaths in Henry's family during the past year.

Henry's parents were never married, and he has had no contact with his biological father. He was raised for the first 12 years of his life by his biological mother who was 16 years old at the time of Henry's birth. Developmental milestones were attained normally, but it is reported that he was born addicted to heroin. It is also alleged that he was sexually abused by a youth in his neighborhood. For several years,

Henry's mother had a common-law husband. The maternal family history is positive for substance abuse. Henry was placed in foster care at the age of 12 after his mother abandoned him.

Henry began to have psychological problems after being exposed to a very traumatic event at the age of nine. He and his ten-year-old aunt found the body of a close family friend. The victim had been decapitated by the common-law husband of Henry's mother. Since that time, he has had chronic problems with early, middle, and terminal insomnia, as well as frequent nightmares and flashbacks. Henry has also been obsessed with killing and being killed and at the age of ten he tried to hang himself. He has also overdosed once on aspirin and once on his brother's imipramine.

Henry has been tested with the WISC-R, revealing a full scale score of 92, a verbal score of 82, and a performance score of 106, with abilities testing finding a developmental reading and arithmetic disorder. He has been involved in several fights and was adjudicated guilty of breaking and entering two years before the present evaluation.

Henry was evaluated at a residential treatment facility. He was administered the Bender Visual Motor Gestalt Test, the

Rorschach Inkblot Technique, the Thematic Apperception Test, and the MMPI–A. The Bender revealed markedly poor visual perceptual function with Koppitz system errors of rotation, angulation, and collision. The projective personality tests found no evidence of a psychosis but indicated that Henry was quite impulsive. Pervasive underlying depression was suggested as well as probable suicidal ideation. He was limited in his social interests and appeared to have strong oppositional tendencies. He was likely to be guarded and mistrustful with possible paranoid ideation.

MMPI–A INTERPRETATION
Profile Validity

Henry produced a valid MMPI–A profile although there are several indications of unusual responding in his validity scales. He failed to respond to three of the test items, but there was no consistent content theme in the omitted items. Henry's scores on the consistency scales of the MMPI–A indicate that he had a moderate tendency toward inconsistent true responding. However, his level of acquiescence was not sufficient to invalidate the resulting test scores. Henry's scores on F and its subscales indicate that he acknowledged having a number of psychological problems and that he did not appear to be exaggerating or over-reporting in responding to the test items.

Overall, Henry's MMPI–A validity scales indicate that he produced a valid profile, that he had a moderate tendency toward acquiescence that did not invalidate the resulting profile, and that he acknowledged having some problems without appearing to exaggerate or over–report their severity.

Current Level of Adjustment

Henry's MMPI–A profile indicates that he is experiencing a considerable degree of psychological distress at this time. He produced elevated scores on six of the eight original clinical scales and on eleven of the fifteen content scales. Thus, Henry reports experiencing adjustment difficulties in a number of different areas of functioning. His moderate elevation on the F scale is also consistent with indications that Henry is experiencing psychological problems at this time. The pattern of scores on the clinical scales does not point to one particular area of dysfunction. However, the content scales suggest a predominantly externalizing pattern of problems.

Symptoms and Traits

Henry produced primary elevations on clinical scales 4 and 6. This pattern of scores indicates that he tends to be angry, resentful, and argumentative. Henry likely acts out aggressively toward others and may have recurring problems with the law. He likely makes excessive demands for attention on others, and he tends to become resentful when demands are placed upon him. He tends to be suspicious of the motives of others, and he is likely to avoid forming close emotional attachments. Henry rejects responsibility for his problems and tends to project blame onto others. He is likely to be viewed by others as aggressive, hostile, and bitter. He is at increased risk for having a substance-use problem. Research indicates that adolescents who produce elevated scores on Scale 4 in clinical settings are more likely than others to have a history of having been sexually abused.

Examination of Henry's scores on the subscales for Scale 4 indicates that his elevation on this scale stems primarily from the endorsement of items describing familial discord and dysfunction. A similar examination of the subscales for Scale 6 indicates that Henry believes that others seek to harm him and that he is hypersensitive to perceived criticism by others.

Henry produced significant elevations on a number of additional clinical scales. His elevation on Scale 9 indicates that Henry tends to show poor judgment and poor impulse control. He may also be distractible. Henry may have an unrealistically positive self–view and he may create an initial impression of being outgoing and gregarious. He is likely to be self–centered and self–indulgent and may demonstrate emotional lability.

Henry's elevation on Scale 7 indicates that he is experiencing some anxiety and emotional discomfort at this time. This may be secondary to the legal difficulties he presently faces. Research indicates that adolescent boys who produce elevated scores on this scale may be at greater risk for having been sexually abused in the past.

Examination of Henry's scores on the relevant subscales indicates that his elevation on Scale 8 stems primarily from feelings of social alienation, his belief that he has gotten a raw deal from life, and his general mistrust of others and inability to form meaningful emotional ties. Finally, Henry's elevation on Scale 1 indicates that he is somewhat preoccupied with physical health concerns.

Henry's scores on the MMPI–A content scales provide additional information regarding his present psychological makeup and functioning. He produced a highly elevated score on the Adolescent Negative Treatment Indicators (A–trt) scale, indicating that Henry holds a number of attitudes and beliefs that may interfere with successful psychological intervention. He tends to have difficulties self–disclosing to others, he may mistrust mental-health professionals, and it is likely that he is not highly motivated to receive psychotherapy at this time.

Henry's score on the Adolescent Anger (A–ang) content scale indicates that he has significant anger-control problems, that he likely experiences outbursts of uncontrollable anger, that his mood tends to be irritable, and that he may over–react to seemingly minor provocation. Research indicates that adolescent boys who produce elevated scores on this scale in clinical settings are more likely than others to have a history of having been sexually abused.

Henry generated an elevated score on the Adolescent Conduct Problems (A–con) scale. This score reflects Henry's tendency toward anti–social acting-out behavior and

a general attitude that it is "OK" to break the law as long as you don't get caught. Adolescents who produce an elevated score on this scale acknowledge engaging in a large number of acting-out behaviors that may result in legal problems. They also tend to blame others for their difficulties. They tend to be entertained by criminal behavior and do not blame people for taking advantage of others. His elevation on the Adolescent School Problems (A–sch) scale suggests that Henry's acting-out tendencies carry over to the school setting and that he is likely, as a result, to have significant disciplinary problems as well as poor academic performance.

His elevated score on the Adolescent Alienation (A–aln) scale indicates that Henry reports experiencing considerable emotional distance from others. He believes that no one, not even members of his family, understands or cares about him and that he is not liked by his peers. Henry views others as a source of threat, rather than support, and he is unlikely to be able to form deep emotional ties. He is also likely to have significant difficulties opening up to others, a tendency that may account for a substantial portion of his elevation on A–trt.

Henry produced an elevated score on the Adolescent Family Problems (A–fam) scale. This score indicates that he perceives his family as conflictual and unloving, that he does not believe that he can turn to members of his family for love or emotional support, and that he likely feels distant and alienated from his family. Henry's score on this scale must be considered in the context of his having been abandoned by his biological father at birth and by his mother at the age 12. It may also be part of a more general tendency toward interpersonal alienation captured by Henry's elevated score on A–aln.

Henry also generated an elevated score on Adolescent Bizarre Mentation (A–biz). Although his level of elevation on this scale is not sufficient to suggest the presence of psychotic symptoms, it does indicate that Henry possesses a large number of rather unusual thoughts and beliefs. Other indicators on the MMPI–A suggest that these may be focussed on paranoid ideation regarding the motives of others whom Henry may believe are enemies who seek to harm him.

Henry's elevated score on the Adolescent Anxiety (A–anx) scale, consistent with his score on Scale 7, indicates a moderate level of anxiety and psychological distress or discomfort that may be secondary to the legal difficulties that led to his current psychological evaluation. Finally, Henry's relatively elevated score on Adolescent Low Self–Esteem (A–lse) indicates that in spite of an external facade of confidence (suggested by an elevated score on Scale 9), Henry may harbor significant insecurities. This raises the possibility that these insecurities may underlie some of Henry's severe acting-out tendencies as well as his difficulties in establishing meaningful emotional ties.

Overall, Henry's MMPI–A profile suggests that he engages in substantial acting-out behavior, that he is interpersonally hostile and aggressive, that he views others as a source of threat rather than support, and that he likely has great difficulties trusting others and forming meaningful emotional attachments. Henry feels distant from most people, including members of his family — which he perceives as a source of conflict and strife. He believes that he cannot be loved by others and that there are people who seek to harm him. Henry believes that he gets a raw deal from life and he tends to project blame for many of his problems onto others. He becomes very resentful when he perceives that others are placing unreasonable demands upon him. He has significant difficulties controlling his anger and has a generally irritable mood. Henry possesses a number of unusual beliefs and thoughts, many of which may be related to his tendency to perceive threat from others. His acting-out behaviors are likely to occur across various settings, including at school where he is likely to have substantial disciplinary problems and poor academic per-

formance. Finally, Henry may be experiencing some anxiety at this time which may be secondary to his current legal difficulties.

Diagnostic Suggestions

Henry's MMPI–A profile is suggestive of a number of diagnoses that should be explored and receive further consideration. The possibility of a severe conduct disorder is clearly indicated by Henry's MMPI–A profile.

Other diagnostic possibilities include a paranoid, schizoid, or schizotypal personality disorder. The nature of Henry's unusual thoughts and beliefs that led to his elevated score on A–biz should be explored further to help in making this determination. The possibility that Henry's score on this scale may, in part, reflect drug–related experiences needs also to be explored. Along these lines, Henry produced a highly elevated score on the Revised MacAndrew (MAC–R) scale. This indicates the strong possibility that Henry possesses personality characteristics such as sensation seeking and a propensity to risk taking that place him at increased risk for developing a substance-use problem.

Treatment Recommendations

A behavioral management program based on strict contingencies should be considered for addressing Henry's substantial acting-out problems and tendencies. Social-skills training, aimed at helping Henry to feel more socially competent, may also be indicated. Individual therapy aimed at understanding and addressing Henry's underlying insecurities should also be considered.

Henry produced elevations on three MMPI–A scales, 4, 7, and A–ang, that are correlated with a history of having been sexually abused. As has been emphasized throughout this book, such elevations, in themselves, are by no means sufficient to indicate that an adolescent has indeed been abused sexually in the past. They are best viewed as red flags that call the attention of the therapist to the *possibility* of sexual abuse, and indicate that it may be fruitful to explore this possibility at some point during the therapy. In Henry's case, there were indications from background information that he was indeed sexually abused by a neighbor boy several years older than himself over a prolonged period of time in the past. The therapist may wish to examine what role such abuse may have played in Henry's difficulties in forming emotional attachments.

His highly elevated score on A–trt indicates the likelihood that his therapist will encounter substantial obstacles and resistance from Henry. His general distrust of people and his anti–social attitudes are likely to pose substantial challenge to Henry's therapist. However, these tendencies should not be interpreted to suggest that Henry is unlikely to benefit from therapy. Rather, they are best viewed as sources of difficulty that should be expected and addressed in Henry's treatment program.

OUTCOME

Henry was diagnosed as evidencing Conduct Disorder, Adolescent Onset Type, Post Traumatic Stress Disorder, as well as Developmental Reading and Developmental Arithmetic Disorder, by history. He was placed in a residential setting and initially was quite distant from his peers. He gradually began to join them in structured recreational therapy but remained distant from staff. He was seen in individual therapy with a focus on cognitive control of his emotions, impulse control, and anger management. In art therapy, he was able to begin to express his feelings of trauma and gain a sense of control. He was placed in special education with tutoring. Henry was subsequently placed in a treatment foster home with follow–up outpatient therapy.

CASE 8
"HENRY"

MMPI-A*

Extended Score Report

ID Number 8

Henry

Male

Age 14

5/07/93

CASE 8
"HENRY"

MMPI-A BASIC SCALES PROFILE

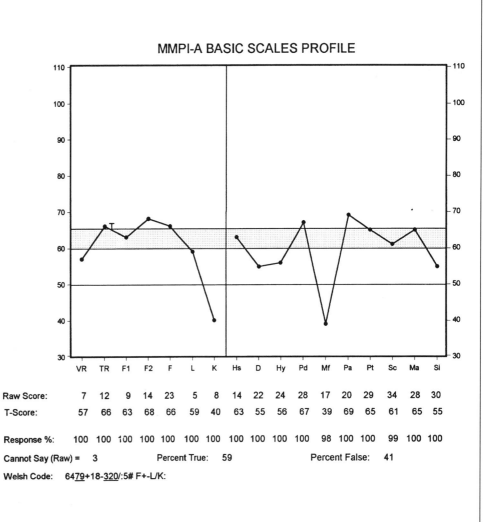

	VR	TR	F1	F2	F	L	K	Hs	D	Hy	Pd	Mf	Pa	Pt	Sc	Ma	Si
Raw Score:	7	12	9	14	23	5	8	14	22	24	28	17	20	29	34	28	30
T-Score:	57	66	63	68	66	59	40	63	55	56	67	39	69	65	61	65	55
Response %:	100	100	100	100	100	100	100	100	100	100	100	98	100	100	99	100	100

Cannot Say (Raw) =   3   Percent True: 59   Percent False: 41

Welsh Code: 64<u>79</u>+18-<u>320</u>/:5# F+-L/K:

CASE 8
"HENRY"

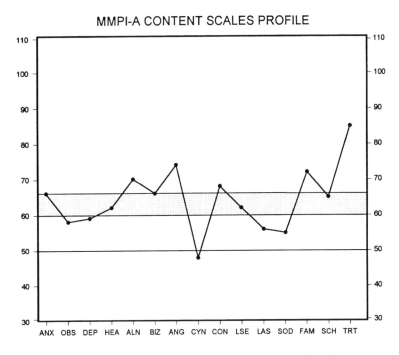

MMPI-A CONTENT SCALES PROFILE

	ANX	OBS	DEP	HEA	ALN	BIZ	ANG	CYN	CON	LSE	LAS	SOD	FAM	SCH	TRT
Raw Score:	14	10	12	15	12	9	14	13	16	9	8	11	22	11	20
T-Score:	66	58	59	62	70	66	74	48	68	62	56	55	72	65	85
Response %:	100	100	100	100	95	100	100	100	100	100	94	96	100	95	100

SUPPLEMENTARY SCORE REPORT

	Raw Score	T Score	Resp %
MacAndrew Alcoholism-Revised (MAC-R)	33	77	100
Alcohol/Drug Problem Acknowledgement (ACK)	6	59	100
Alcohol/Drug Problem Proneness (PRO)	22	62	100
Immaturity Scale (IMM)	28	73	100
Anxiety (A)	25	65	100
Repression (R)	15	54	100

Depression Subscales (Harris-Lingoes)

	Raw Score	T Score	Resp %
Subjective Depression (D1)	14	63	100
Psychomotor Retardation (D2)	3	41	100
Physical Malfunctioning (D3)	5	62	100
Mental Dullness (D4)	5	56	100
Brooding (D5)	4	56	100

Hysteria Subscales (Harris-Lingoes)

	Raw Score	T Score	Resp %
Denial of Social Anxiety (Hy1)	0	32	100
Need for Affection (Hy2)	5	50	100
Lassitude-Malaise (Hy3)	6	58	100
Somatic Complaints (Hy4)	9	67	100
Inhibition of Aggression (Hy5)	2	44	100

Psychopathic Deviate Subscales (Harris-Lingoes)

	Raw Score	T Score	Resp %
Familial Discord (Pd1)	7	69	100
Authority Problems (Pd2)	5	60	100
Social Imperturbability (Pd3)	2	42	100
Social Alienation (Pd4)	6	55	100
Self-Alienation (Pd5)	6	57	100

Paranoia Subscales (Harris-Lingoes)

	Raw Score	T Score	Resp %
Persecutory Ideas (Pa1)	9	68	100
Poignancy (Pa2)	5	61	100
Naivete (Pa3)	2	40	100

CASE 8
"HENRY"

Schizophrenia Subscales (Harris-Lingoes)

Social Alienation (Sc1)	12	68	100
Emotional Alienation (Sc2)	4	59	100
Lack of Ego Mastery, Cognitive (Sc3)	5	59	100
Lack of Ego Mastery, Conative (Sc4)	6	57	100
Lack of Ego Mastery, Defective Inhibition (Sc5)	4	53	100
Bizarre Sensory Experiences (Sc6)	7	56	100

Hypomania Subscales (Harris-Lingoes)

Amorality (Ma1)	6	73	100
Psychomotor Acceleration (Ma2)	7	52	100
Imperturbability (Ma3)	4	55	100
Ego Inflation (Ma4)	5	53	100

Social Introversion Subscales (Ben-Porath, Hostetler, Butcher, & Graham)

Shyness / Self-Consciousness (Si1)	9	59	100
Social Avoidance (Si2)	2	47	100
Alienation--Self and Others (Si3)	11	60	100

Uniform T scores are used for Hs, D, Hy, Pd, Pa, Pt, Sc, Ma, and the Content Scales; all other
MMPI-A scales use linear T scores.

OMITTED ITEMS

The following items were omitted by the client. It may be helpful to discuss these item omissions with this individual to determine the reason for non-compliance with test instructions.

251. I wish I were not bothered by thoughts about sex.
450. I get along with most people.
464. Others tell me that I am lazy.

End of Report

SUGGESTED ITEMS FOR FOLLOW-UP

ALCOHOL/DRUG PROBLEMS

342. I can express my true feelings only when I drink. (T)

458. I sometimes get into fights when drinking. (T)

SUICIDAL BEHAVIORS

177. I sometimes think about killing myself. (T)

FAMILY PROBLEMS

440. I have spent nights away from home when my parents did not know where I was. (T)

CASE 9
"ISAIAH"

FORENSIC ASSESSMENT OF A PARANOID–DELUSIONAL YOUNGSTER WITH VERY POOR IMPULSE CONTROL

BACKGROUND

Isaiah, a 16-year-old, Caucasian male, was admitted to a closed residential setting for evaluation and treatment recommendations by the juvenile court. He had been placed in a detention center where he was reported to have been experiencing auditory and visual hallucinations. He was, as well, combative and exhibited self-injurious behavior. He had a history of elopement from open residential treatment settings.

Isaiah and a twin sister were born when their father and mother were 16 and 17 years old, respectively. The parents were married at the time of the childrens' birth. They divorced when the twins were one year old. No contact has taken place since then with the father. The twins were born two months premature.

Isaiah had a birth weight of three pounds and a heart murmur. He was epileptic and was treated since age one with phenobarbital. When he was seven, he was kidnapped from his elementary school and sexually abused by an older male. He was found by his family in a dumpster. At age 14, he was involved in a serious automobile accident in a stolen car driven by a friend. Isaiah sustained severe head trauma and a crushed leg. He was comatose for four days. Since then, he reported hearing voices telling him to harm himself and experiencing visual hallucinations. His speech, since the accident, has been slurred. He has been placed in Severe Behavioral Handicap classes since first grade. He has a history of polysubstance abuse since age 11. Five years before this evaluation, Isaiah was tested with the WISC–R and found to have a verbal score of 73, a performance score of 106, and a full scale IQ score of 87.

Upon admission to the closed residential facility, Isaiah was administered a Rorschach, Human Figures Drawings, and a Bender Visual Motor Gestalt Test. The Rorschach was significant for low productivity and extreme concreteness of thought. His response style was impulsive and erratic. There were strong indications of emotional discomfort and lability. The record was similar to organically impaired populations. The HFD suggested concreteness and impulsivity. The Bender Gestalt found Koppitz errors of rotation and marked distortion.

MMPI–A INTERPRETATION
Profile Validity

Isaiah produced a valid MMPI–A profile. He responded to all of the test items and provided a coherent and consistent set of responses. His score on TRIN indicates a moderate tendency toward inconsistent true responding. However, his level of acquiescence was not sufficient to raise concerns about the validity of the resulting test scores. Isaiah did produce elevated scores on the F scales, most notably F_1. His scores on these scales indicate that Isaiah acknowledged experiencing significant psychological problems at this time. However, they do not indicate a tendency on his part to exaggerate or over–report his problems. Overall, this is an interpretable profile and Isaiah's cooperation with the MMPI–A can be viewed as a positive indication of his involvement with the evaluation.

Current Level of Adjustment

Isaiah's MMPI–A profile indicates that he is experiencing considerable psychological problems at this time. He produced elevated scores on numerous MMPI–A clinical scales, and his pattern of elevation was characterized by a positive slope, with the greatest elevation occurring on the right–hand side of the profile. This indicates that Isaiah is undergoing considerable psychological turmoil and suggests the possibility that he is having difficulties with reality testing. Examination of the content scales reveals a similar pattern. Although Isaiah does not produce a large number of elevations on the content scales, his substantial elevation on the Adolescent Bizarre Mentation (A–biz) scale suggests the possibility of severe psychological disturbance. Secondary elevations on clinical scales 2 and 7 also indicate that Isaiah is experiencing considerable psychological distress at this time.

Symptoms and Traits

Isaiah's most prominently elevated scale on the clinical profile is Scale 6. Isaiah's score on this scale is highly elevated. Coupled with his pattern of elevation on the relevant subscales, this elevation indicates a substantial likelihood that he is experiencing paranoid delusional thinking at this time. Isaiah likely believes that he has ene-

mies who wish to harm him, and he may interpret benign statements or actions as posing a threat to his safety and wellbeing. He likely experiences a great deal of anger and resentment, and projection is likely to be his primary defense mechanism. Thus, Isaiah may be inclined to attribute to others the hostile, aggressive impulses that he feels toward them. He is also likely to be hypersensitive to perceived slights and criticism.

Isaiah produced secondary elevation on Scale 4, indicating a tendency toward poor impulse control and acting-out behaviors. Thus, Isaiah may be inclined to act upon the delusional fears and beliefs indicated by his elevation on Scale 6. In addition, he likely has substantial academic and disciplinary problems in school, and he may have difficulties incorporating the values and standards of society. Further, Isaiah may be particularly rebellious and hostile toward authority figures. He may have a very low tolerance for frustration and boredom. His elevation on this scale indicates that Isaiah may also be inclined toward the use of alcohol and/or drugs.

Examination of Isaiah's scores on the subscales of Scale 2 indicates that his elevated score on this scale likely reflects a diffuse sense of depression and dysphoric mood. He likely experiences apathy and a general disinterest in activities. He may also be socially withdrawn. As with any case where the possibility of depression is indicated, the potential for suicidal ideation or gestures needs to be considered. This is particularly true of profiles indicative of poor impulse control. Examination of the list of Suggested Items for Follow–up indicates that Isaiah does indeed acknowledge some suicidal ideation.

Isaiah's elevation on Scale 7 indicates that he is experiencing some psychological discomfort at this time. As indicated by his pattern of scores on the relevant subscales, Isaiah's moderate elevation on Scale 8 appears to reflect his feeling that he is losing control over his thoughts and emotions, that he is unable to control his impulses, and that he may be subjected to very unusual sensory experiences, possibly including hallucinations. The possible role that drug use may play in these experiences needs to be considered.

Isaiah's moderately elevated score on Scale 9 indicates that he is restless and agitated, demonstrates irresponsible behavior and poor impulse control, and, once again, suggests the possibility that Isaiah may be inclined to act out impulsively upon his paranoid beliefs and suspicions. This score also raises the possibility that Isaiah may engage in alcohol and/or drug use.

Finally, examination of the relevant subscales indicates that Isaiah's elevated score on Scale 0 does *not* necessarily reflect social introversion or discomfort in this case. Rather, it is the alienation component of this scale that appears to be driving this moderate elevation. This interpretation is supported by Isaiah's average score on the content scale Adolescent Social Discomfort (A–sod) and his elevated score on the content scale Adolescent Alienation (A–aln).

Isaiah's scores on the MMPI–A content scales indicate that his acting-out behaviors may be expressed most prominently in school. His elevated score on the Adolescent School Problems (A–sch) scale indicates that Isaiah reported experiencing a large number of disciplinary and academic problems at school. He is likely to have difficulties interacting with both teachers and peers, and, given his poor impulse control, Isaiah may be inclined toward becoming involved in physical altercations with peers.

Isaiah's elevated score on Adolescent Conduct Problems (A–con) indicates that his acting-out problems are by no means limited to the school setting. He acknowledges engaging in a wide range of anti–social behaviors including stealing and lying, and he is likely to be generally oppositional. Isaiah may try to blame others for his problems, and he is very reluctant to assume responsibility for any of his difficulties.

Isaiah's elevated score on A–biz indicates that he reports having a large number of very unusual thoughts and experiences that may include psychotic symptoms and behav-

iors. He may experience delusional thinking (in light of his elevation on Scale 6 this would be primarily of a paranoid, persecutory nature), as well as hallucinations. The possible role of drugs in these experiences needs to be examined. But Isaiah's elevated score on this scale indicates that he is experiencing very serious and unusual symptoms of psychological disorder at this time.

Isaiah also produced an elevated score on A–aln, indicating that he experiences considerable emotional distance from others and that he finds it very difficult to form meaningful emotional ties. Isaiah likely believes that others do not care about him, and he therefore makes no attempts to get close to people and he does not allow others to get close to him.

Isaiah produced a moderately elevated score on Adolescent Low Self–Esteem (A–lse), indicating that he tends to hold a rather negative, depreciatory self–view. Isaiah likely has little or no confidence in his ability to succeed in life, and he likely perceives himself as a failure. Isaiah's moderately elevated score on Adolescent Negative Treatment Indicators (A–trt) most likely reflects his general mistrust of others, particularly those whom he perceives as being in positions of authority, including mental-health professionals.

Overall, Isaiah's MMPI–A profiles indicate that he tends to be very suspicious of others and that he may experience paranoid delusional thinking. He may also experience other psychotic symptoms including, possibly, hallucinations. Isaiah views others as threatening, and he may be inclined to act on these perceptions. He has very poor impulse control and is prone toward aggressive, acting-out behavior. These tendencies are likely to cause Isaiah to experience considerable psychological difficulties, and they may result in his getting into trouble with the law. When this occurs, Isaiah is likely to blame others for his problems, and he is not likely to assume any responsibility for his own actions. He is particularly suspicious of individuals in positions of authority. His most severe acting-out behaviors may occur in school, and he is likely to have very significant disciplinary and academic problems in that environment. However, Isaiah's acting-out behaviors are not limited to school and would tend to generalize across settings. It is very likely that he has already had legal difficulties, or, if not, that he may have such difficulties in the not too distant future.

Isaiah's scores also indicate that he has difficulties forming close social ties. These difficulties are likely not the product of social anxiety or discomfort. Rather, they most likely reflect Isaiah's general tendency to mistrust others and keep them at a distance. Isaiah likely does not feel very strong emotions. However, he does report experiencing some dysphoric affect and anxiety at this time. These experiences may be secondary to his presently being placed in a locked unit with very strict supervision and control.

Diagnostic Suggestions

Isaiah's MMPI–A profile indicates the possibility of a psychotic disorder, including paranoid schizophrenia, a delusional disorder, or atypical psychosis. Background information indicates that Isaiah has fairly recently sustained a significant closed head injury, that he continues to manifest overt signs of neuropsychological dysfunction, and that the emergence of psychotic symptoms coincides with the injury. Therefore, the possibility of an organically based psychotic disorder should be considered. A diagnosis of conduct disorder should also be considered based on Isaiah's MMPI–A profile.

Isaiah's MMPI–A profile also suggests a strong likelihood that he has a substance-use problem He produced a highly elevated score on the Revised MacAndrew (MAC–R) scale, indicating that he possesses a large number of personality characteristics related to sensation-seeking and risk-taking that place him at risk for developing a substance use problem. He also produced a moderately elevated score on the Alcohol/Drug Problem Proneness (PRO) scale, indicating further the possibility that

Isaiah has personality characteristics placing him at risk for substance-use problems. Isaiah's elevated score on the Alcohol/Drug problem Acknowledgment scale indicates that he admits abusing alcohol and possibly also drugs. As indicated earlier in this book, although a non–elevated score on this scale cannot be used to rule out the possibility of a substance-use problem, an elevated score on this scale is a very strong indicator of such problems. Examination of the list of Suggested Items for Follow–up shows that Isaiah did, indeed, endorse a number of MMPI–A items indicative of problematic substance use.

Treatment Recommendations

Isaiah's MMPI–A profile suggests the need for an immediate psychiatric evaluation to determine whether he may benefit from psychotropic medication. In addition, a highly structured behavioral contingency program may be indicated to attempt to control Isaiah's acting-out tendencies. In light of his difficulties with reality testing and impulse control, a highly structured and secure setting may be the most effective environment for treating Isaiah's current severe psychological problems. In addition, Isaiah acknowledges experiencing some suicidal ideation at this time, indicating the need for a careful examination of his potential for suicide and supporting further the desirability of placing Isaiah in a highly structured and closely supervised environment.

OUTCOME

Isaiah's diagnoses were Organic Hallucinosis and Organic Mood Disorder, Depressed as well as a Conduct Disorder, Solitary Aggressive Type and Polysubstance Abuse. He was recommended for placement in a secure setting. After a psychiatric evaluation, he was started on Tegratol, Thorazine, and Clonidine. He was placed in structured group therapy and a fairly basic cognitive therapy. Shortly after admission, when refused privileges after not earning them through the day, Isaiah became quite combative. He injured two staff members and broke out a plexiglass reinforced window with a chair. He escaped and broke into a construction trailer. He was apprehended and his probation was revoked. He was placed in the juvenile justice system in a facility for emotionally disturbed juvenile offenders.

CASE 9
"ISAIAH"

MMPI-A*

Extended Score Report

ID Number 9

Isaiah

Male

Age 16

6/10/93

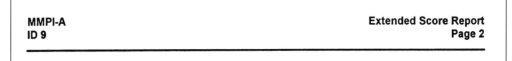

MMPI-A
ID 9

Extended Score Report
Page 2

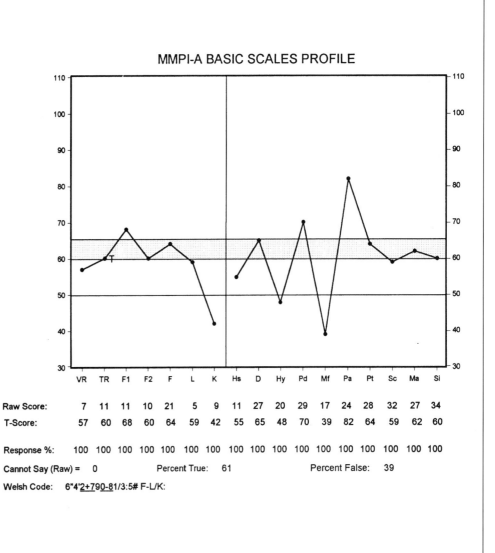

MMPI-A BASIC SCALES PROFILE

	VR	TR	F1	F2	F	L	K	Hs	D	Hy	Pd	Mf	Pa	Pt	Sc	Ma	Si
Raw Score:	7	11	11	10	21	5	9	11	27	20	29	17	24	28	32	27	34
T-Score:	57	60	68	60	64	59	42	55	65	48	70	39	82	64	59	62	60

Response %: 100 100 100 100 100 100 100 100 100 100 100 100 100 100 100 100 100

Cannot Say (Raw) = 0   Percent True: 61   Percent False: 39

Welsh Code: 6"4'2+790-81/3:5# F-L/K:

CASE 9
"ISAIAH"

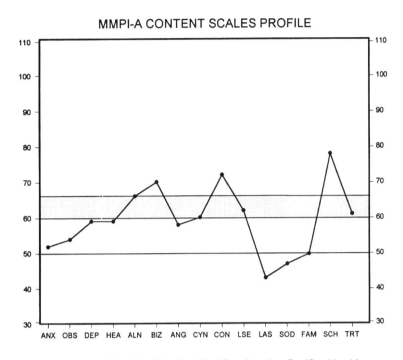

MMPI-A CONTENT SCALES PROFILE

	ANX	OBS	DEP	HEA	ALN	BIZ	ANG	CYN	CON	LSE	LAS	SOD	FAM	SCH	TRT
Raw Score:	9	9	12	14	11	10	11	17	17	9	4	7	12	14	14
T-Score:	52	54	59	59	66	70	58	60	72	62	43	47	50	78	61
Response %:	100	100	100	100	100	100	100	100	100	100	100	100	100	100	100

SUPPLEMENTARY SCORE REPORT

	Raw Score	T Score	Resp %
MacAndrew Alcoholism-Revised (MAC-R)	31	72	100
Alcohol/Drug Problem Acknowledgement (ACK)	8	67	100
Alcohol/Drug Problem Proneness (PRO)	21	60	100
Immaturity Scale (IMM)	21	62	100
Anxiety (A)	21	59	100
Repression (R)	14	51	100

Depression Subscales (Harris-Lingoes)

	Raw Score	T Score	Resp %
Subjective Depression (D1)	14	63	100
Psychomotor Retardation (D2)	7	61	100
Physical Malfunctioning (D3)	5	62	100
Mental Dullness (D4)	7	64	100
Brooding (D5)	6	66	100

Hysteria Subscales (Harris-Lingoes)

	Raw Score	T Score	Resp %
Denial of Social Anxiety (Hy1)	1	38	100
Need for Affection (Hy2)	6	54	100
Lassitude-Malaise (Hy3)	4	50	100
Somatic Complaints (Hy4)	6	57	100
Inhibition of Aggression (Hy5)	3	51	100

Psychopathic Deviate Subscales (Harris-Lingoes)

	Raw Score	T Score	Resp %
Familial Discord (Pd1)	4	53	100
Authority Problems (Pd2)	6	67	100
Social Imperturbability (Pd3)	1	35	100
Social Alienation (Pd4)	8	65	100
Self-Alienation (Pd5)	10	73	100

Paranoia Subscales (Harris-Lingoes)

	Raw Score	T Score	Resp %
Persecutory Ideas (Pa1)	14	86	100
Poignancy (Pa2)	6	67	100
Naivete (Pa3)	3	45	100

CASE 9
"ISAIAH"

Schizophrenia Subscales (Harris-Lingoes)

Social Alienation (Sc1)	8	56	100
Emotional Alienation (Sc2)	3	54	100
Lack of Ego Mastery, Cognitive (Sc3)	7	68	100
Lack of Ego Mastery, Conative (Sc4)	3	46	100
Lack of Ego Mastery, Defective Inhibition (Sc5)	7	67	100
Bizarre Sensory Experiences (Sc6)	10	65	100

Hypomania Subscales (Harris-Lingoes)

Amorality (Ma1)	4	59	100
Psychomotor Acceleration (Ma2)	9	62	100
Imperturbability (Ma3)	3	49	100
Ego Inflation (Ma4)	5	53	100

Social Introversion Subscales (Ben-Porath, Hostetler, Butcher, & Graham)

Shyness / Self-Consciousness (Si1)	6	49	100
Social Avoidance (Si2)	3	52	100
Alienation--Self and Others (Si3)	13	66	100

Uniform T scores are used for Hs, D, Hy, Pd, Pa, Pt, Sc, Ma, and the Content Scales; all other MMPI-A scales use linear T scores.

End of Report

SUGGESTED ITEMS FOR FOLLOW-UP

ALCOHOL/DRUG PROBLEMS

144. I have a problem with alcohol or drugs. (T)

161. I have had periods in which I carried on activities without knowing later what I had been doing. (T)

247. I have used alcohol excessively. (T)

458. I sometimes get into fights when drinking. (T)

474. People often tell me I have a problem with drinking too much. (T)

SUICIDAL BEHAVIORS

177. I sometimes think about killing myself. (T)

FAMILY PROBLEMS

440. I have spent nights away from home when my parents did not know where I was. (T)

460. I have never run away from home. (F)

CASE 10

"JULIE"

A MOOD DISORDER
WITH PSYCHOTIC FEATURES

BACKGROUND

Julie is a 16-year-old, Caucasian female who was transferred to a closed residential treatment facility from an inpatient psychiatric hospital. She resides with her parents and three older brothers. The family lives in a middle-class area and the parents are very religious.

Julie was delivered by C–section at 7.5 months without complications and achieved developmental milestones in a normal sequence. At age five, she was raped by a neighborhood man who was a convicted child molester. The rape was discovered when she was found outside the house bleeding profusely. After this incident, Julie began wearing several layers of clothing, even in warm weather.

At age ten, Julie witnessed a small boy being killed by a school bus in front of her house. Following this, she refused to ride school buses and had difficulty crossing the street. At age 11, she was, herself, struck by a car and received crushing injuries to the tibia and fibula. At age 12, her mother was diagnosed as suffering from multiple sclerosis. When Julie was 15, she suffered a knee injury in soccer that required surgical repair and ended her ability to participate in sports, in which she had been quite

active. Both of Julie's parents have a history of treatment for depression, with the mother having one suicide attempt by overdose in the 1970s.

Julie's recent psychiatric hospitalization began upon referral from her outpatient therapist with precipitating symptoms of depression, weight loss, variations in eating, decreased sleep, and psychomotor slowing. She confided to a school counselor that she was suicidal. She was hospitalized briefly, released, and, upon returning home, cut her arm quite deeply with a razor blade. She was returned to the hospital and referred to a closed residential treatment facility for further evaluation and treatment.

One year before the current evaluation, Julie had been given a WISC–III with a verbal score of 88; a performance score of 83 and a full scale score of 84. At that time, projective testing using the Rorschach and Figure Drawings found evidence of significant depression, low self-esteem, and a perception by Julie that the only solution to her problems was death.

At the time of admission evaluation, she was administered the MMPI–A, the Beck Depression Inventory (BDI), and the Beck Hopelessness (BHS) scale. The BDI score was 38, which is in the significantly depressed range, and the BHS score was 19, reflecting considerable feelings of hopelessness and likely suicidal ideation.

MMPI–A INTERPRETATION
Profile Validity

Julie's scores on the MMPI–A validity scales raise several questions regarding the validity of her profile. She responded to all but one of the MMPI–A items and produced a consistent and coherent set of responses. Her T score of 40 on VRIN indicates that Julie was particularly careful and meticulous in responding to the test items, a positive sign of her involvement with the evaluation. Her score of 59 on TRIN indicates a very slight tendency toward inconsistent false responding that in no way affects the validity of the remaining MMPI–A scales. She produced an elevated score on the F scale and a particularly elevated score on the subscale F_1.

Whenever an adolescent produces an elevated score on the F scale, the interpreter's task is to differentiate between three non–mutually–exclusive possible reasons for elevation on this scale: random responding, severe psychological disorder, and over–reporting of symptoms. Random responding can easily be ruled out in this case because of Julie's low score on VRIN. We know from background information that Julie is presently experiencing severe psychological problems that are consistent with her level of elevation on the F scales. Thus, in this case, Julie's elevated score on F and its subscales is most reasonably interpreted as reflecting the severe psychological distress with which she is presently contending, and random responding and over–reporting of symptoms are ruled out.

The discrepancy between Julie's scores on F_1 and F_2 indicates that she tended to produce more deviant responses to the first part than to the second part of the MMPI–A booklet. It is important to realize that *deviance*, here, is defined statistically based on item-endorsement percentages. Examination of Julie's raw scores on F_1 and F_2 indicates that she endorsed 13 of the 33 F_1 items and 14 of the 33 F_2 items in the deviant direction. Yet, her T score on F_1 is considerably higher than her T score on F_2. This is possible because, on average, F_1 items were less frequently endorsed by the MMPI–A normative sample than are F_2 items. Thus, a comparison of Julie's raw scores on these subscales would be highly misleading. F_1/F_2 comparisons should always be conducted at the T-score, not raw-score level. A pattern of T scores like the one in this case is found frequently in MMPI–A profiles characterized by endorsement of psychotic symptoms, most of which appear within the first half of the booklet and therefore fall on F_1 more than on F_2. Thus, Julie's pattern of scores on F_1 and F_2 does not indicate invalid responding to one part of the booklet and is consistent with background information indicating that she is experiencing severe psychological problems.

A final issue to be addressed in Julie's validity scale profile is her elevated score on L (T-score = 70). Because TRIN is only slightly elevated, we can rule out a false response set as a possible cause for this elevation. Elevated scores on L are sometimes produced by adolescents who come from very traditional homes where religious and moral values have been deeply ingrained in the test–taker. In Julie's case, background information indicates that her parents are very religious individuals who have emphasized religious and moral values in the upbringing of their children. This may account for some of her elevation on L. However, this is not likely to account for all of her elevation on this scale.

Thus, it would appear that Julie adopted a somewhat guarded and defensive approach to the test and made an unsophisticated attempt to portray herself in an overly positive light by denying minor faults and shortcomings that most adolescents readily acknowledge. The fact that Julie's score on K is not also elevated indicates that Julie's defensiveness was limited to this type of naive denial of shortcomings. Had she taken an overall defensive approach, we would expect to find little in her clinical scales and virtually no elevation in her content scales. Examination of these scales indicates that this clearly is not the case in Julie's profile. Thus, her defensive responding was very circumscribed, a pattern that is sometimes seen in individuals who are experiencing paranoid delusional thinking.

Overall, then, Julie produced a valid MMPI–A profile. She responded to all but one of the test items and produced a consistent and coherent set of responses. Julie responded in the keyed direction to a large number of infrequently endorsed items, reflecting her present experience of severe and unusual psychological problems. In responding to some of the test items, she was guarded and defensive, adopting a rather unsophisticated test–taking approach in an attempt to portray herself as a highly moral person. In spite of this approach to the MMPI–A, Julie reported a large number of psychological problems and produced an interpretable set of MMPI–A scale scores.

Current Level of Adjustment

Julie's MMPI–A profile indicates that she is experiencing severe psychological problems and turmoil at this time. She produced highly elevated scores on several of the MMPI–A clinical and content scales, and the pattern of her scores on the MMPI–A clinical scales is indicative of possible psychotic symptomatology. This possibility is supported by Julie's highly elevated score on the Adolescent Bizarre Mentation (A–biz) scale. In addition to psychotic symptoms, Julie reports feeling very depressed, and examination of her responses to the list of Suggested Items for Follow–up indicates that she reports having suicidal thoughts at this time. Overall, Julie's MMPI–A profile indicates that she is currently experiencing acute psychological distress.

Symptoms and Traits

Julie's most prominent elevation on the MMPI–A clinical scales is on Scale 6. Her highly elevated score on this scale indicates that Julie is likely experiencing paranoid delusional thinking, she believes that she has enemies who seek to harm her, she is likely

experiencing substantial impairment in her reality testing, and she may show a number of symptoms of a formal thought disorder.

Julie also produced a highly elevated score on Scale 2 of the MMPI–A, indicating that she is presently experiencing a large number of symptoms of a depressive disorder. She reports having a very dysphoric mood, she tends to brood and focus on her perceived shortcomings, and she feels generally lethargic and unable to confront her difficulties. She likely feels apathetic and lacking interest in anything in her life right now. She may feel very guilty about her perceived inadequacies. Julie's level of depression, as reflected in her level of elevation on Scale 2, suggests the possibility that she may be suicidal at this time. As already noted, examination of her responses to the list of Suggested Items for Follow–up indicates that she did indeed endorse MMPI–A items indicative of current suicidal ideation.

Julie's elevation on clinical scale 4 may, at first blush, appear to be suggestive of acting-out problems. However, examination of scores on the relevant subscales indicates that it is predominantly a sense of alienation from herself and others that is responsible for Julie's elevation on this scale. She does not report any substantial conflict with authority figures or with members of her family. A similar pattern is seen in several of Julie's scores on the MMPI–A content scales which indicate that she does not report acting-out behaviors or family problems. However, she does relate a strong sense of emotional alienation.

Examination of the relevant subscales indicates that Julie's elevated score on clinical scale 3 is most likely reflective of a general sense of emotional fatigue, poor appetite, difficulties in concentration, and generally dysphoric affect. She may also have a heightened need for attention. Finally, examination of the relevant subscales indicates that Julie's elevated score on Scale 0 is *not* indicative of social introversion or discomfort. Rather, it too is reflective of Julie's overall sense of emotional and social alienation.

Examination of Julie's scores on the

MMPI–A content scales provides a somewhat different perspective on her current psychological difficulties. Whereas her scores on the clinical scales might be viewed as indicating that Julie's most prominent problems have to do with psychotic symptomatology, with a secondary problem with depression, her scores on the content scales indicate that Julie describes both areas of functioning as equally problematic for her at this time. She produced highly elevated scores on both Adolescent Depression (A–dep) and Adolescent Bizarre Mentation (A–biz). Her elevated score on A–dep indicates that Julie reports feeling very prominent and severe symptoms of depression including dysphoric mood, low drive, self–depreciatory thoughts, and suicidal ideation. She is very dissatisfied with her life and is likely to experience crying spells. Her elevated score on A–biz indicates that Julie reports experiencing a large number of very unusual thoughts and perceptions that may include auditory and visual hallucinations and bizarre delusional beliefs. She likely believes that others are plotting against her and have engaged in various attempts to harm her. Her level of elevation on this scale indicates very poor reality testing.

Julie also produced a highly elevated score on the Adolescent Low Self–Esteem (A–lse) scale. This score indicates that she holds a very negative self-view, that she is lacking in self–confidence and views herself as very unattractive, and that she likely believes that she cannot do anything well. She is likely to be very submissive in interpersonal relationships and does not feel comfortable having to make any decisions for herself. She likely becomes very uncomfortable if people say nice things about her.

Julie also produced an elevated score on the Adolescent Negative Treatment Indicators (A–trt) scale. This score indicates that she reports holding a number of views, attitudes, and beliefs that may interfere with her treatment. She may believe that no one can help her, and she may have a negative view of mental-health professionals.

She may also report having difficulties trusting others and disclosing her problems to them. She may be generally pessimistic about her future, including any treatment that may be offered to her.

Julie generated an elevated score on the Adolescent Anxiety scale (A–anx). This score indicates that she reports feeling a substantial amount of subjective anxiety at this time and that she may generally feel very nervous and tense. Her elevated score on the Adolescent Alienation scale (A–aln), reinforces other indications in Julie's MMPI–A profile that she feels very distant from others, that she is unable to form meaningful emotional ties, and that she generally views others as a source of stress and potential harm, rather than support. Finally, Julie's elevated sore on the Adolescent Obsessiveness (A–obs) scale indicates that she is inclined to engage in obsessive rumination about her problems and likely has considerable difficulties making decisions.

In addition to identifying several areas of severe psychological dysfunction, Julie's scores on the MMPI–A content scales also point to several potential areas of strength. Her average score on the Adolescent School Problems scale (A–sch) indicates that Julie does not view this area of her life as problematic. Background information indicates that, indeed, until her recent hospitalization Julie was excelling in her academic pursuits at school and was not experiencing any disciplinary problems. Her relatively low score on the Adolescent Low Aspirations (A–las) scale indicates similarly that Julie continues to aspire toward academic accomplishments.

Finally, Julie produced a very low score on the Adolescent Family Problems (A–fam) scale. This score indicates that Julie reported a considerably smaller number of family problems than did the average girl in the MMPI–A normative sample. On the face of it, this would identify her family as an important potential source of support for Julie. However, background information indicates that, although intact, Julie's family has experienced considerable conflict and turmoil. Thus, it appears that Julie's circumscribed, naive attempt to portray herself in an overly positive light (see the previous discussion of her elevation on L) may have been focussed primarily on describing an unrealistic, idyllic family life. This issue will be considered further under treatment recommendations.

Overall, Julie's MMPI–A profile indicates that she is experiencing very severe psychological problems at this time. She reports experiencing a number of psychotic symptoms including delusions and hallucinations and is likely to be very paranoid at this time. Concomitantly, Julie reports very severe symptoms of depression, dysphoric affect, lack of drive, many self–depreciatory thoughts and beliefs, and active suicidal ideation. Julie also feels very alienated from others emotionally and does not believe that she is able to form meaningful relationships. She views people as being distant and aloof, and may be viewed similarly by others. She has a very negative opinion of herself and tends to be highly pessimistic about any improvement in her situation. The one area where she continues to function well at this time is at school where she does not report having many problems and where she continues to aspire to achieve academic success. She holds a naive view of her family as loving and caring, and is reluctant to admit or discuss any shortcomings in her family.

Diagnostic Suggestions

Julie's MMPI–A profile provides strong indications that she may be experiencing both a psychotic disorder and a mood disorder. Her highly elevated scores on A–biz and Scale 6 indicate that the possibility of a paranoid schizophrenic disorder, a delusional disorder, or an atypical psychotic disorder should be considered. Her scores also indicate a strong possibility that Julie may be experiencing a major depressive disorder that may be accompanied by psychotic features. A major differential diagnostic issue is whether Julie's psychotic symptoms are independent from, or part

of, a possible mood disorder. The possibility of a schizoaffective disorder needs also to be considered. Julie's very low self–esteem and her suicidal ideation also indicate the possibility of a developing borderline personality disorder. Finally, examination of the MMPI–A list of Suggested Items for Follow–up indicates that Julie reports engaging in some unusual eating patterns that may be indicative of bulimia.

Insofar as the primary referral issue is concerned, Julie's MMPI–A profile is particularly instructive in that it indicates that psychotic symptoms may be playing a more prominent role in her condition than had been known before this evaluation.

Treatment Recommendations

Julie's MMPI–A profile indicates the need for an immediate psychiatric evaluation to determine whether she is in need of psychotropic medication. The diagnostic suggestions indicated by her profile and the severity of the symptoms she reports indicate that she likely will be prescribed medication. Her profile also indicates that Julie continues to be very suicidal at this time, and that she presently needs to be kept under close supervision in a highly structured, therapeutic environment.

Once her condition has stabilized, it will be important to help Julie become engaged in her new environment. Individual therapy aimed at helping Julie challenge her very negative self–view is recommended. Providing Julie with an opportunity to form a warm therapeutic relationship may help her begin to regain some trust in others and in her ability to form meaningful relationships. Participation in group therapy activities may help in accomplishing similar goals.

A careful exploration of Julie's need to portray her family as free of any difficulty and strife may be indicated once her condition has stabilized and improved. Throughout her treatment, Julie's strong academic aspirations should be encouraged and reinforced.

OUTCOME

Julie was admitted to the facility's intensive-care residential center. Her diagnoses were Major Depression, Recurrent with mood congruent psychotic features; Post Traumatic Stress Disorder, and developing Borderline Personality traits. A potential eating disorder was also suggested. She was prescribed both anti–depressive and anti–psychotic medication.

During her initial stay at the facility, Julie was seen as continuing to be depressed. She reported hearing a voice that she described as "no good" which tells her she should either harm herself or die. She indicated that she does act upon that voice. Julie initially was quite guarded and suspicious of others. She would become episodically and unpredictably assaultive or would attempt to harm herself, generally by attempting to cut herself or bang her head against a wall. Following these incidents, she would appear to dissociate with generally little recall of the event. Of spe-

cial note were Julie's academic skills. In spite of her many emotional problems, she continued to excel academically at the facility's school.

Julie gradually became involved in individual therapy, initially with an orientation toward building a relationship and enhancing a sense of safety. Thereafter, cognitive behavioral strategies were introduced in the areas of response to her trauma, depression, self control, and anger management. Julie was also seen in a therapy group which included a focus on sexually traumatized girls. Family therapy was initiated.

Julie was eventually returned home and placed in a partial hospitalization program. Her course there was variable, as at times she would decompensate to the extent of requiring brief stabilization at the intensive-care center. In time, however, she was able to manage her emotions to the extent that stabilization needs decreased substantially. She was eventually returned to her home school, where she remains.

MMPI-A*

Extended Score Report

ID Number 10

Julie

Female

Age 16

4/29/93

MMPI-A BASIC SCALES PROFILE

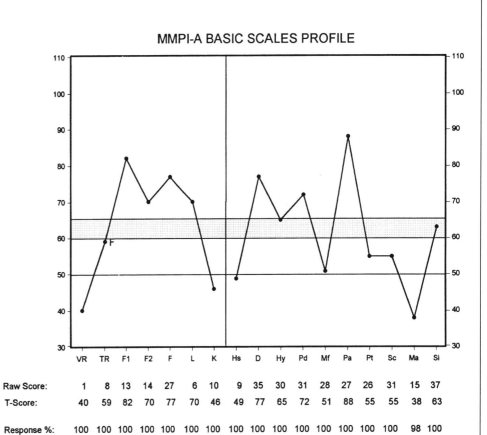

	VR	TR	F1	F2	F	L	K	Hs	D	Hy	Pd	Mf	Pa	Pt	Sc	Ma	Si
Raw Score:	1	8	13	14	27	6	10	9	35	30	31	28	27	26	31	15	37
T-Score:	40	59	82	70	77	70	46	49	77	65	72	51	88	55	55	38	63
Response %:	100	100	100	100	100	100	100	100	100	100	100	100	100	100	100	98	100

Cannot Say (Raw) =   1   Percent True: 53   Percent False: 47

Welsh Code: 6"24'3+0-785/1:9# FL'+-/K:

CASE 10
"JULIE"

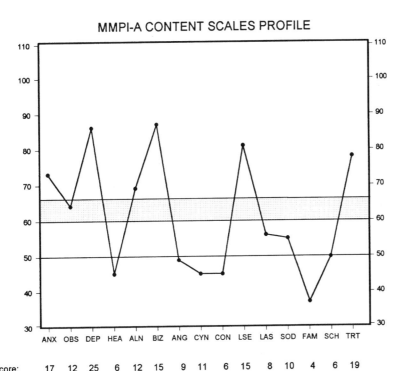

MMPI-A CONTENT SCALES PROFILE

	ANX	OBS	DEP	HEA	ALN	BIZ	ANG	CYN	CON	LSE	LAS	SOD	FAM	SCH	TRT
Raw Score:	17	12	25	6	12	15	9	11	6	15	8	10	4	6	19
T-Score:	73	64	86	45	69	87	49	45	45	81	56	55	37	50	78
Response %:	100	100	100	100	100	100	100	100	100	100	100	100	100	100	100

SUPPLEMENTARY SCORE REPORT

	Raw Score	T Score	Resp %
MacAndrew Alcoholism-Revised (MAC-R)	18	46	100
Alcohol/Drug Problem Acknowledgement (ACK)	2	43	100
Alcohol/Drug Problem Proneness (PRO)	13	41	100
Immaturity Scale (IMM)	18	60	100
Anxiety (A)	29	66	100
Repression (R)	16	58	100
Depression Subscales (Harris-Lingoes)			
Subjective Depression (D1)	23	78	100
Psychomotor Retardation (D2)	8	67	100
Physical Malfunctioning (D3)	5	58	100
Mental Dullness (D4)	8	66	100
Brooding (D5)	9	74	100
Hysteria Subscales (Harris-Lingoes)			
Denial of Social Anxiety (Hy1)	3	48	100
Need for Affection (Hy2)	7	59	100
Lassitude-Malaise (Hy3)	9	65	100
Somatic Complaints (Hy4)	5	50	100
Inhibition of Aggression (Hy5)	4	58	100
Psychopathic Deviate Subscales (Harris-Lingoes)			
Familial Discord (Pd1)	3	45	100
Authority Problems (Pd2)	3	52	100
Social Imperturbability (Pd3)	2	43	100
Social Alienation (Pd4)	11	75	100
Self-Alienation (Pd5)	11	75	100
Paranoia Subscales (Harris-Lingoes)			
Persecutory Ideas (Pa1)	17	98	100
Poignancy (Pa2)	3	46	100
Naivete (Pa3)	7	66	100

CASE 10
"JULIE"

Schizophrenia Subscales (Harris-Lingoes)

Social Alienation (Sc1)	11	64	100
Emotional Alienation (Sc2)	5	65	100
Lack of Ego Mastery, Cognitive (Sc3)	7	67	100
Lack of Ego Mastery, Conative (Sc4)	11	75	100
Lack of Ego Mastery, Defective Inhibition (Sc5)	4	49	100
Bizarre Sensory Experiences (Sc6)	4	46	100

Hypomania Subscales (Harris-Lingoes)

Amorality (Ma1)	3	55	100
Psychomotor Acceleration (Ma2)	5	39	100
Imperturbability (Ma3)	0	31	100
Ego Inflation (Ma4)	3	41	89

Social Introversion Subscales (Ben-Porath, Hostetler, Butcher, & Graham)

Shyness / Self-Consciousness (Si1)	7	52	100
Social Avoidance (Si2)	2	51	100
Alienation--Self and Others (Si3)	13	63	100

Uniform T scores are used for Hs, D, Hy, Pd, Pa, Pt, Sc, Ma, and the Content Scales; all other
MMPI-A scales use linear T scores.

OMITTED ITEMS

The following items were omitted by the client. It may be helpful to discuss these item omissions with this individual to determine the reason for non-compliance with test instructions.

199. I have been inspired to a program of life based on duty which I have since carefully followed.

End of Report

SUGGESTED ITEMS FOR FOLLOW-UP

EATING DISORDER SYMPTOMS

108. Sometimes I make myself throw up after eating so I won't gain weight. (T)

SUICIDAL BEHAVIORS

177. I sometimes think about killing myself. (T)

283. Most of the time I wish I were dead. (T)

CASE 11
"KYLE"

AN EARLY INDICATION OF
PENDING PSYCHOTIC DECOMPENSATION

BACKGROUND

Kyle is a 14-year-old, Caucasian male who was admitted to the intensive-care center upon referral from a children's services board. The history indicated that his parents divorced when he was 10 years old. His father remarried and disowned Kyle after learning that his name was not on the birth certificate. The youth was repeatedly sexually abused by his mother and her boyfriend. The mother is reported to have been heavily involved in substance abuse. He was removed from the home at age 12.

Beginning at age 11, Kyle began to show severe behavioral difficulties and was placed in a Severe Behavioral Handicap program at school. He began to have juvenile court involvement with charges of receiving stolen property, resisting arrest, theft, assault, criminal damaging, and runaway. He had a series of temporary foster-home placements and ran away from each of them.

Presently, Kyle is placed at the residential treatment center by the juvenile court as an alternative to placement in the correctional system. A psychological evaluation conducted for the court indicated diagnoses of Conduct Disorder and Dysthymia.

Upon admission to the intensive-care center, Kyle was initially fairly quiet and withdrawn. However, after a few days he began to evidence behavioral difficulties in which he would become assaultive. In the admission interview, he was seen as denying depression but admitting to thoughts of cutting his wrists when he was arrested by the police on the theft charge. He admitted cutting his wrists at age 13 but would not give details. He did acknowledge a feeling of "being watched."

MMPI–A INTERPRETATION
Profile Validity

Kyle's scores on the MMPI–A validity scales raise questions about the validity of his profile. He responded to all of the test items. He produced a relatively low score on VRIN, indicating that he was able to process and respond relevantly to the test items and that he was particularly careful and cautious in his approach to the test. In particular, Kyle made an effort to avoid contradicting himself in responding to the test items. His moderately elevated score on TRIN indicates that Kyle did provide some inconsistent "true" responses. However, his level of acquiescence would not be expected to have an effect on the validity of his scores on the remaining MMPI–A scales.

Kyle produced very elevated scores on scale F and its subscales. His pattern of scores on F_1 and F_2 indicates that he produced a similar level of unusual responding to the first and second halves of the MMPI–A booklet.

As already discussed with reference to several other cases in this book, when confronted with an elevated score on F the test-interpreter needs to differentiate between three possible non–mutually–exclusive reasons for elevation on this scale: random responding, severe psychological problems, and over–reporting of symptoms. In this case, we can rule out random responding based on Kyle's low score on VRIN. From background data, we know that Kyle has had severe behavioral control problems and that he has recently been diagnosed as having a dysthymic mood disorder. Neither of these conditions would be sufficient to cause the level of elevation seen in Kyle's score on F. Because Kyle had just been admitted to the intensive care center when he completed the MMPI–A, clinical observations of his condition were unavailable to the interpreter. Thus, the absence of any clinical or background indications of severe psychological disturbance suggests the possibility of over–reporting of symptoms. Examination of Kyle's pattern of scores on the MMPI–A clinical and content scales also indicates the likelihood that he may have over–reported or exaggerated his difficulties. His pattern of elevation on the content scales is particularly diffuse, and thus indicative of over–reporting of symptoms.

Based on the analysis so far, it is apparent that Kyle has over–reported some of his psychological problems. However, it is important to keep in mind that, based upon background information, Kyle does have some genuine problems. Thus, it would be inappropriate to conclude on the basis of the MMPI–A that Kyle is malingering. Rather, Kyle's approach to the MMPI–A may best be viewed as an exaggeration and over–elaboration of existing problems, in what has traditionally been termed "A cry for help."

If one uses this conceptualization, one concludes that Kyle is likely to be experiencing significant psychological distress at this time and, in response to difficulties in understanding and describing his problems, he has opted to complain of a wide array of symptoms and problems. Kyle's low scores on L and K which, given his score on TRIN, cannot be attributed to a response set, are consistent with the view that Kyle is overwhelmed by his difficulties at this time.

Because of Kyle's approach to the MMPI–A, his scores on the clinical and content scales are likely to overestimate the severity of some of his problems. However, the pattern, rather than absolute elevation, of these scores can still provide useful interpretive information. Thus, his scores on the MMPI–A clinical, content, and supplementary scales can be interpreted with caution.

Current Level of Adjustment

Kyle's MMPI–A profile indicates that he is experiencing considerable psychological distress and turmoil at this time. He may feel that he is losing control, and he may be overwhelmed and unable to cope with his current difficulties.

Indications of Kyle's severe distress include his combination of elevation on F and low scores on L and K, his very high elevations on the clinical scales, and in particular the content scales, and his exceptionally high elevation on the content scale Adolescent Bizarre Mentation (A–biz). Kyle's score on this scale indicates that he reports experiencing a large number of severe, psychotic symptoms. Because of issues identified above under profile validity, Kyle's highly elevated score on this scale cannot be taken at face value to suggest that he is indeed experiencing *many* psychotic symptoms at this time. However, it remains possible that he is presently suffering from *some* psychotic symptoms that are causing him to feel very scared and confused.

Another indication of Kyle's severe level of distress is the positive slope of his scores on the MMPI–A clinical scales, where most of the elevation (with the exception of Scale

4) is found on the right–hand side of the profile. This pattern is also suggestive of the possibility that Kyle may be experiencing some psychotic symptoms at this time. Finally, examination of the list of Suggested Items for Follow–up indicates that Kyle reports current suicidal ideation.

Overall, then, Kyle's profile indicates that he is presently experiencing very severe psychological problems that likely have left him feeling overwhelmed and ineffective.

Symptoms and Traits

For reasons outlined in the discussion of the validity of Kyle's profile, a scale-by-scale interpretive approach is inappropriate in this case because of Kyle's apparent over–reporting of symptoms. However, an examination of the pattern of his scores on the MMPI–A scales can yield some general statements about his current difficulties. Kyle's most highly elevated MMPI–A score is on Adolescent Bizarre Mentation (A–biz). This indicates that Kyle reports experiencing severe psychotic symptoms including delusions and hallucinations. His highly elevated scores on clinical scales 6 and 8 are consistent with this interpretation. Kyle's pattern of scores on the subscales for Scale 6 indicates that he may be experiencing paranoid delusions. Because of his over–reporting tendency, it is not possible to determine weather Kyle is indeed experiencing psychotic symptoms at this time. Background information does not indicate any history of psychotic symptoms and clinical observations have yet to be performed at the time of testing. However, the possibility exists that Kyle may be in the early stages of a psychotic condition and may, as a result, feel very confused and overwhelmed at this time.

Another possibility that should be considered is that some of the symptoms Kyle reports may be the product of drug and alcohol use. He produced very elevated scores on all three MMPI–A substance-use scales and he acknowledges readily that he has problems in this area (see his responses to several of the Suggested Items for Follow–up).

Kyle's MMPI–A scores also indicate the likelihood of severe acting-out problems. His elevations on clinical scales 4 and 9 indicate a propensity toward impulsive, irresponsible, acting-out behaviors and that Kyle may have problems managing and controlling his anger. These difficulties likely result in poor academic performance and disciplinary problems in school. This is also indicated by his highly elevated scores on the content scales Adolescent Anger (A–ang), Adolescent Conduct Problems (A–con), and Adolescent School Problems (A–sch).

As indicated by elevations on the content scales Adolescent Alienation (A–aln) and Adolescent Cynicism (A–cyn), Kyle reports holding a very cynical view of others. He believes that people are not to be trusted and that they look out only for their own interests. He also finds it very difficult to form and maintain meaningful emotional ties with others. As indicated by his score on Adolescent Family Problems (A–fam), Kyle's estrangement from others includes members of his family. Examination of the list of Suggested Items for Follow–up indicates that Kyle reports having gotten many beatings and having frequently run away from home.

A final area of concern based on Kyle's MMPI–A profile is his current mood state. Although not as elevated as his scores on some of the other scales, Kyle's scores on clinical scales 2 and 7 and content scales Adolescent Anxiety (A–anx) and Adolescent Depression (A–dep) suggest that he may feel very depressed and anxious at this time. As already noted, Kyle's responses to several MMPI–A items indicate that he currently is experiencing suicidal ideation.

Overall, Kyle's MMPI–A profile indicates that he reports experiencing very severe psychotic symptoms at this time including hallucinations and delusions. The latter may take on a paranoid flavor. The veracity of these symptoms is in question owing to indications that Kyle over–reported his problems. However, the possibility that he may be experiencing the early stages of a psychotic condition cannot be ruled out at this time. Kyle's scores also show that he has severe acting-out problems, very poor impulse control and judgment, and that he is likely, as a result, to have legal problems. He feels very alienated from and distrusting of others and he reports a very conflictual family life. Kyle also reports having a depressed mood and feeling very anxious.

Diagnostic Suggestions

Because of Kyle's approach to the MMPI–A his scores on the test can provide only very tenuous suggestions insofar as possible diagnoses are concerned. First, as already discussed, the possibility that Kyle *may* be experiencing initial stages of decompensation associated with a psychotic disorder needs to be considered. Another possibility is that Kyle's previously diagnosed dysthymic disorder has now worsened, and he may be experiencing a major depressive episode with psychotic features. His MMPI–A profile indicates that Kyle continues to report symptoms of depression and anxiety at this time.

Kyle's profile indicates very strongly that he has a severe conduct disorder. His scores on the Revised MacAndrew (MAC) and Alcohol/Drug Problem Proneness (PRO) scales indicate that Kyle possesses personality characteristic such as sensation-seeking, risk–taking, and a susceptibility to the negative influences of peers, which place him at considerable risk for developing a substance-use problem. His score on the Alcohol/Drug Problems Acknowledgment (ACK) scale, indicates that Kyle acknowledges having substantial problems in this area.

Treatment Recommendations

Kyle's MMPI–A profile indicates the need to place him under close observation. He has reported suicidal ideation and has very poor impulse control. Thus, he is at substantial risk for a suicidal gesture or attempt. Further, Kyle feels very overwhelmed at this time, and he may be experiencing the initial symptoms of a psychotic disorder. An immediate referral for a psychiatric examination to determine Kyle's need for medication is indicated. Once his condition has stabilized, he should be referred for individual therapy. A contingency–based behavioral approach to managing Kyle's severe acting-out tendencies may be attempted. Providing Kyle with an opportunity to form a warm therapeutic relationship may also help him to overcome his apparently deep–rooted mistrust of and alienation from others.

OUTCOME

One day after the administration of the MMPI–A, Kyle became floridly psychotic on the unit. He actively hallucinated, reporting hearing voices, and he became highly agitated, extremely combative, and uncommunicative. Staff had been put on alert based on the MMPI–A data and were able to respond in a supportive and protective manner to prevent harm to Kyle or others. Since that time, he has been treated with anti–psychotic medication. He is involved in art therapy, group therapy, substance-abuse treatment, and individual therapy focussing on relationships, reality testing, and cognitive regulation of emotions. He is also in a focussed treatment group for traumatized youth.

Kyle has shown a generally good response to treatment but occasionally he has episodic periods of acting-out in an aggressive fashion. His current diagnoses include Major Depression with Psychotic Features, Post Traumatic Stress Disorder, Conduct Disorder, and Polysubstance Abuse. The discharge plans call for placement in a specialized treatment foster home with wrap-around services and placement in a partial hospitalization program.

MMPI-A*

Extended Score Report

ID Number 11

Kyle

Male

Age 14

8/24/93

CASE 11
"KYLE"

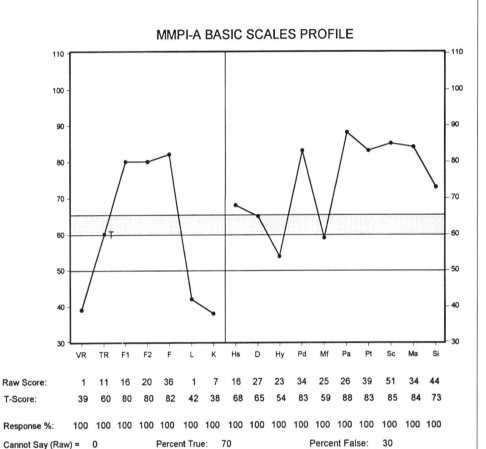

MMPI-A BASIC SCALES PROFILE

	VR	TR	F1	F2	F	L	K	Hs	D	Hy	Pd	Mf	Pa	Pt	Sc	Ma	Si
Raw Score:	1	11	16	20	36	1	7	16	27	23	34	25	26	39	51	34	44
T-Score:	39	60	80	80	82	42	38	68	65	54	83	59	88	83	85	84	73

Response %: 100 100 100 100 100 100 100 100 100 100 100 100 100 100 100 100 100

Cannot Say (Raw) = 0   Percent True: 70   Percent False: 30

Welsh Code: 68947"0'12+-53/ F'''+-/L:K#

CASE 11
"KYLE"

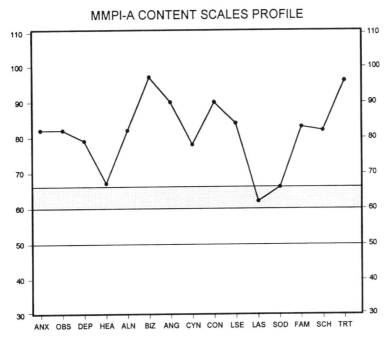

MMPI-A CONTENT SCALES PROFILE

	ANX	OBS	DEP	HEA	ALN	BIZ	ANG	CYN	CON	LSE	LAS	SOD	FAM	SCH	TRT
Raw Score:	19	15	20	17	15	17	17	21	22	14	9	15	26	15	23
T-Score:	82	82	79	67	82	97	90	78	90	84	62	66	83	82	96
Response %:	100	100	100	100	100	100	100	100	100	100	100	100	100	100	100

SUPPLEMENTARY SCORE REPORT

	Raw Score	T Score	Resp %
MacAndrew Alcoholism-Revised (MAC-R)	32	75	100
Alcohol/Drug Problem Acknowledgement (ACK)	13	87	100
Alcohol/Drug Problem Proneness (PRO)	27	74	100
Immaturity Scale (IMM)	32	79	100
Anxiety (A)	29	70	100
Repression (R)	12	47	100
Depression Subscales (Harris-Lingoes)			
Subjective Depression (D1)	20	77	100
Psychomotor Retardation (D2)	4	46	100
Physical Malfunctioning (D3)	6	68	100
Mental Dullness (D4)	8	68	100
Brooding (D5)	8	76	100
Hysteria Subscales (Harris-Lingoes)			
Denial of Social Anxiety (Hy1)	0	32	100
Need for Affection (Hy2)	2	37	100
Lassitude-Malaise (Hy3)	10	74	100
Somatic Complaints (Hy4)	8	64	100
Inhibition of Aggression (Hy5)	1	36	100
Psychopathic Deviate Subscales (Harris-Lingoes)			
Familial Discord (Pd1)	6	64	100
Authority Problems (Pd2)	6	67	100
Social Imperturbability (Pd3)	1	35	100
Social Alienation (Pd4)	10	74	100
Self-Alienation (Pd5)	11	78	100
Paranoia Subscales (Harris-Lingoes)			
Persecutory Ideas (Pa1)	14	86	100
Poignancy (Pa2)	6	67	100
Naivete (Pa3)	2	40	100

CASE 11
"KYLE"

Schizophrenia Subscales (Harris-Lingoes)

Social Alienation (Sc1)	14	74	100
Emotional Alienation (Sc2)	7	76	100
Lack of Ego Mastery, Cognitive (Sc3)	7	68	100
Lack of Ego Mastery, Conative (Sc4)	8	65	100
Lack of Ego Mastery, Defective Inhibition (Sc5)	10	82	100
Bizarre Sensory Experiences (Sc6)	14	77	100

Hypomania Subscales (Harris-Lingoes)

Amorality (Ma1)	6	73	100
Psychomotor Acceleration (Ma2)	9	62	100
Imperturbability (Ma3)	3	49	100
Ego Inflation (Ma4)	6	58	100

Social Introversion Subscales (Ben-Porath, Hostetler, Butcher, & Graham)

Shyness / Self-Consciousness (Si1)	10	62	100
Social Avoidance (Si2)	5	62	100
Alienation--Self and Others (Si3)	17	77	100

Uniform T scores are used for Hs, D, Hy, Pd, Pa, Pt, Sc, Ma, and the Content Scales; all other
MMPI-A scales use linear T scores.

End of Report

SUGGESTED ITEMS FOR FOLLOW-UP

ALCOHOL/DRUG PROBLEMS

144. I have a problem with alcohol or drugs. (T)

161. I have had periods in which I carried on activities without knowing later what I had been doing. (T)

247. I have used alcohol excessively. (T)

342. I can express my true feelings only when I drink. (T)

431. Talking over problems and worries with someone is often more helpful than taking drugs or medicines. (F)

458. I sometimes get into fights when drinking. (T)

467. I enjoy using marijuana. (T)

474. People often tell me I have a problem with drinking too much. (T)

SUICIDAL BEHAVIORS

177. I sometimes think about killing myself. (T)

283. Most of the time I wish I were dead. (T)

FAMILY PROBLEMS

366. I have gotten many beatings. (T)

440. I have spent nights away from home when my parents did not know where I was. (T)

460. I have never run away from home. (F)

CASE 12

"LARRY"

INDICATIONS OF EARLY STAGES OF A THOUGHT DISORDER

BACKGROUND

Larry is an 18–year–old, single Caucasian male who was readmitted to a secure residential treatment facility following two years of open residential care and nine months of partial hospitalization treatment. Before readmission, he had been discharged from partial hospitalization by his placing agency against clinical advice and had been transferred to a group home. While there, he sexually assaulted another client who was confined to a wheelchair.

Larry was born to parents who were both markedly dysfunctional, with a history of mental illness and substance abuse. He was physically abused as an infant and removed from the home. He was adopted at age two and was sexually abused in the adoptive home. At age four, he was sexually abused by his biological uncle. In elementary school, he was reported to evidence severe behavioral difficulties and also began cross–dressing. He was placed on Ritalin at that time for hyperactivity. During middle childhood and early adolescence, Larry was primarily seen as being introverted. At age 16, he attempted to poison his adoptive parents with lighter fluid when they discovered a bra in his bedroom.

Medically, it is reported that Larry was born with a collapsed trachea and that he has had allergies all of his life. There is no reported history of head trauma, coma, serious illnesses, or major surgeries. There is no record of a significant substance-abuse history. Larry was placed in Severe Behavioral Handicap classes in middle school and never completed high school.

In residential treatment, Larry's course of care was quite variable. He frequently alienated himself from peers owing to his very poor social skills. He would evidence explosive temper outbursts. He was extremely immature and attention-seeking. He continued to compulsively cross-dress and frequently propositioned other youth.

During his diagnostic interview following readmission, Larry appeared much younger than his stated age. His gait and posture were non remarkable. He was right–hand dominant. There were no overt indications of gross or fine motor dysfunction. His speech was generally pressured, immature in tone and normal in volume. There were no indications of loosening of associations, flight of ideas, or tangentiality. His verbalizations were occasionally unusual, but, for the most part, they were highly concrete. Larry's social skills appeared quite poor and he presented with a considerable need for approval. He attempted all testing tasks requested of him but tended to give up quite easily when he became challenged. His approach to problem solving was a non-systematic, trial and error approach.

Larry presented with a slightly expansive and labile affect to a stated anxious and depressed mood. He denied any history of hallucinations or dissociative experiences and there were no present indications of perceptual abnormalities. There were some indications of paranoid ideation and his thinking tended to be illogical, unrealistic, and egocentric. He denied current phobias but his cross dressing behavior was described in a somewhat obsessional and compulsive manner. He indicated current depression specific to his legal circumstances with disturbances in his sleep, as well as an increased appetite. He reported his health to be intact. Larry denied current suicidal ideation, was future oriented, had no specific suicidal plans, and could identify supports in his environment. He denied thoughts of harming others. He did report current anxiety, again specific to his present circumstances.

Larry was oriented to time, place, and person. His long-term, short-term, and immediate recall functions were intact. His recall of digits was six forward and four reversed. He was able to name the four most recent presidents. He was not able to interpret proverbs and had considerable difficulty identifying similarities between related objects. His insight and judgment were markedly below age expectations.

Larry was administered a battery of diagnostic psychological tests including the WAIS–R, Bender Visual Motor Gestalt Test, House Tree Person Technique, Beck Depression Inventory, Beck Hopelessness Scale, and the MMPI–A. He was found to have a WAIS–R verbal IQ of 88, a performance IQ of 86 and a full scale IQ of 86. The Bender record was analyzed using the Koppitz system and yielded mild errors of rotation, angulation, and integration. The projective drawings suggested a markedly

poor self-image and likely withdrawal into fantasy to avoid conflict. The record also suggested primitive emotional development. The Rorschach was found to be similar to records associated with markedly unusual thinking and a probable thought disorder. Larry's thinking was suggested to be often illogical, over-personalized, and egocentric. He appeared to be depressed and anxious with poor cognitive controls over his emotions. A tendency for acting out of conflicts, limited social judgment, and limited social understanding was also suggested. Possible sexual conflicts were also suggested by the record. The Beck Depression Inventory was found to be indicative of clinically significant depression and the Beck Hopelessness scale suggested a risk of suicidal ideation.

MMPI–A INTERPRETATION
Profile Validity

Larry produced a valid MMPI–A profile. He responded to all but one of the test items, and his scores on the consistency scales indicate that he provided a coherent and consistent set of responses. He had moderately elevated scores on F and its subscales, and his scores on F_1 and F_2 did not indicate any qualitative change in his approach to the test between the first and second halves of the MMPI–A booklet. Larry's overall elevation on F does not indicate any over–reporting of problems. His score on L is within the average range, and his low score on K indicates that Larry may be feeling somewhat overwhelmed at this time.

Overall, Larry's test–taking approach was open and cooperative. This can be viewed as a positive indication of his involvement with the evaluation.

Current Level of Adjustment

Larry's MMPI–A profile indicates that he is experiencing considerable psychological distress at this time. He is likely to have a chronic pattern of maladjustment with some current exacerbation of symptoms. Larry's scores on the clinical scales of the MMPI–A form a positive slope, with most of the elevation on the right side of the profile and at considerable levels of elevation. This pattern indicates a chronic pattern of maladjustment that may be characterized by psychotic symptoms. His level of elevation on Scale 7 and on content scales Adolescent Anxiety (A–anx) and Adolescent Depression (A–dep) indicates that Larry is likely experiencing acute psychological distress at this time. His very low score on K indicates that he may be feeling overwhelmed and unable to cope with his current difficulties.

Symptoms and Traits

Larry's MMPI–A profile indicates that he is experiencing acute anxiety at this time. His elevation on Scale 7 indicates that he likely feels tense and nervous, is inclined toward obsessive rumination, and may be plagued by insecurities, and feelings of guilt and self–doubt. This interpretation is supported by his score on the content scale Adolescent Anxiety (A–anx), which indicates that Larry reports having many subjective symptoms of anxiety, and his score on Adolescent Obsessiveness (A–obs), which indicates that he is currently worried and preoccupied, and that he likely has difficulties making decisions because of his obsessive tendencies.

Larry also produced substantial elevations on clinical scales 6 and 8. Examination of the subscales for Scale 6 indicates that his elevation on that scale is driven primarily by persecutory ideation and secondarily by a hyper–sensitivity to perceived criticism. Larry likely views others as threatening and overly critical of him, he likely harbors strong feelings of anger and resentment toward others, he tends to project blame for his difficulties onto others, and he may be manifesting delusional symptoms of a thought disorder.

Larry's elevation on Scale 8 and his pattern of scores on its subscales indicate the possibility that he may be exhibiting symptoms of a thought disorder. He may presently be confused and disorganized and may be withdrawn and socially isolated. Larry's elevation on this scale suggests fur-

ther that he tends to be nonconforming, and possibly socially deviant. Adolescents who produce elevations on this scale tend to have strong feelings of inferiority, incompetence, and low self–esteem.

Larry also produced elevated scores on clinical scales 2 and 0. Examination of the relevant subscales of Scale 2 indicates that Larry may have a depressed mood at this time, and that he is prone to sulk and brood about his problems. His pattern of scores on the subscales for Scale 0 indicates that Larry tends to be overly shy and self–conscious, and suggests that he feels very alienated from himself and others at this time.

Larry's scores on the MMPI–A content scales provide additional and clarifying information regarding the interpretations suggested by his scores on the clinical scales. As already mentioned, Larry's content scale profile indicates that he is very anxious and distressed at this time. In addition, his elevated score on the Adolescent Depression (A–dep) scale indicates a greater level of depression than had been suggested by Larry's score on Scale 2. His score on A–dep indicates that Larry presently experiences substantial symptoms of depression including a dysphoric mood, a lack of drive, self–depreciatory beliefs, and that he may have some suicidal ideation. Examination of the list of Suggested Items for follow–up confirms that Larry does express some suicidal ideation at this time.

Larry also produced an elevated score on Adolescent Bizarre Mentation (A–biz), indicating that he reported a relatively large number of unusual thoughts and experiences. These may include paranoid delusional beliefs as well as other symptoms of a thought disorder. Because Larry's scores on the substance abuse scales do not provide any suggestion of a problem in that area, it is not likely that his unusual thoughts and experiences are the product of drug use. However, this should be considered further based on background and other extra–test data. Although substantially elevated, Larry's score on A–biz is not as high as is seen in cases where adolescents are experiencing floridly psychotic symptoms. Nevertheless, his score on this scale does indicate that he tends to hold very unusual thoughts and beliefs.

One of Larry's highest scores on the MMPI–A content scales is on Adolescent Anger (A–ang). His elevation on this scale indicates that Larry acknowledges having serious anger-control problems. He tends to feel very irritable and is easily frustrated, and responds to these feelings with overt outbursts of anger. Adolescents who produce similar elevations on this scale are likely to have a history of assaultive behavior. Larry also produced an elevated score on the Adolescent Cynicism (A–cyn) scale. His score on this scale indicates that Larry tends to be very cynical and suspicious of the motives of others, he believes that most people would hurt others just to get ahead, and he likely feels that it is safer to trust no one other than himself.

Larry also generated an elevated score on Adolescent Low Aspirations (A–las), indicating that he does not have a very optimistic view of his prospects and that he has presently given up attempting to prepare himself for the future. He is presently disinterested in academic pursuits. Larry's elevated score on the Adolescent Low Self-Esteem (A–lse) scale supports indications in the clinical scales that he tends to have a very negative self–view. His moderately elevated score on Adolescent Alienation (A–aln) confirms indications that Larry views the world as a source of threat and that he likely has difficulties forming warm emotional ties.

Overall, Larry's MMPI–A profile indicates that he presently shows a combination of acute distress and long–standing patterns of chronic maladjustment. He is presently very anxious and concerned, he tends to obsess and brood over his difficulties and may be feeling debilitated by his anxiety. Some of these feelings may be the result of his current legal problems. Larry also reports feeling very depressed at this time and he acknowledges having some suicidal thoughts.

Larry reports some unusual thought processes. He may experience paranoid delusional thinking, and he may hold some odd beliefs. He believes that others seek to harm him and he is overly sensitive to perceived criticism. Larry views others as a source of threat and danger, he is likely unable to form emotional ties with others. He also tends to hold a very negative self–view and he is likely preoccupied with his self–perceived failures. Presently, Larry appears to feel very pessimistic about the future and he may have given up hope of ever achieving any success.

Diagnostic Suggestions

Larry's profile indicates a number of diagnostic possibilities that merit further examination. Because of his elevation on scales 6, 8, and A–biz, the possibility of a formal thought disorder needs to be considered. The likelihood of a full–blown psychotic disorder is somewhat counter–indicated by Larry's *relatively* moderate scores on A–biz and F. Adolescents who experience symptoms of schizophrenia, for example, tend to score higher than Larry on these two scales. The possibility of a delusional disorder, a schizoid personality disorder, or schizotypal personality disorder are all indicated by Larry's scores on these scales.

Other elevations on Larry's MMPI–A profile indicate the possibility of an anxiety and/or mood disorder. The possibility of an obsessive-compulsive disorder is suggested by elevations on Scale 7, A–anx, and A–obs, and the possibility of a depressive disorder is indicated by elevations on Scale 2 and A–dep. Given Larry's current legal problems, it may also be that these elevations reflect the symptoms of an adjustment disorder with mixed emotional features.

Treatment Recommendations

The possibility of a thought disorder indicates that Larry should be referred for a psychiatric evaluation to determine his need for psychotropic medication. His current suicidal ideation indicates the need for a careful examination to determine Larry's risk for harming himself. Individual therapy is indicated to help Larry deal with his present emotional upheaval and to assist him in developing a more positive self–image and to acquire social skills.

His elevated score on Adolescent Negative Treatment Indicators (A–trt) indicates that he possesses attitudes and beliefs that may interfere with treatment. Specifically, Larry may feel pessimistic about the possibility that anyone can help him and he may have significant difficulties opening up to others. It is important to alert the therapist to these possibilities so that she or he might design appropriate confidence–building interventions.

OUTCOME

Larry was given the diagnoses Post Traumatic Stress Disorder, Delayed Onset; Attention Deficit Disorder, Residual; Gender Identity Disturbance of Adolescence; and Schizotypal Personality Disorder. His depression and anxiety were viewed as manifestations of a delayed PTSD which is the result of several traumatic experiences he endured as a child. Examination of his thought processes indicated a propensity toward odd and unusual thoughts and beliefs, but no signs of a formal thought disorder. Following this evaluation, Larry was brought to trial and placed in a sexual offender treatment program.

CASE 12
"LARRY"

MMPI-A*

Extended Score Report

ID Number 12

Larry

Male

Age 18

5/16/94

MMPI-A
ID 12

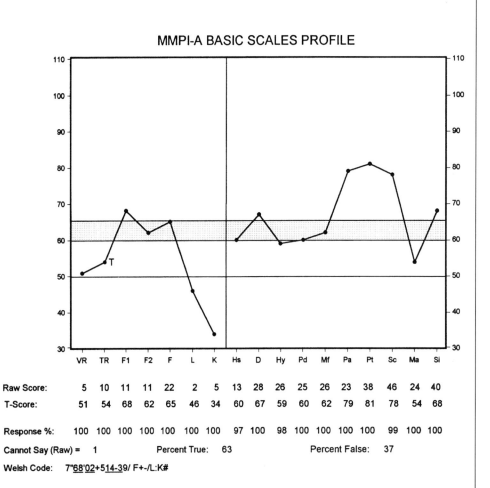

MMPI-A BASIC SCALES PROFILE

	VR	TR	F1	F2	F	L	K	Hs	D	Hy	Pd	Mf	Pa	Pt	Sc	Ma	Si
Raw Score:	5	10	11	11	22	2	5	13	28	26	25	26	23	38	46	24	40
T-Score:	51	54	68	62	65	46	34	60	67	59	60	62	79	81	78	54	68
Response %:	100	100	100	100	100	100	100	97	100	98	100	100	100	100	99	100	100

Cannot Say (Raw) = 1   Percent True: 63   Percent False: 37

Welsh Code: 7"68'02+514-39/ F+-/L:K#

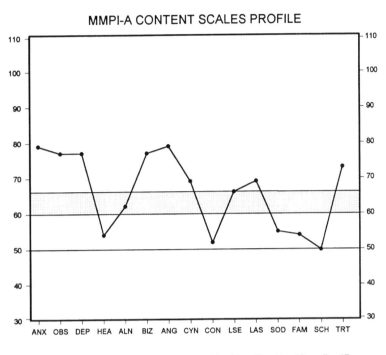

MMPI-A CONTENT SCALES PROFILE

	ANX	OBS	DEP	HEA	ALN	BIZ	ANG	CYN	CON	LSE	LAS	SOD	FAM	SCH	TRT
Raw Score:	18	14	19	11	10	12	15	19	11	10	10	11	15	7	17
T-Score:	79	77	77	54	62	77	79	69	52	66	69	55	54	50	73
Response %:	100	100	100	97	100	100	100	100	100	100	100	100	100	100	100

SUPPLEMENTARY SCORE REPORT

	Raw Score	T Score	Resp %
MacAndrew Alcoholism-Revised (MAC-R)	17	41	100
Alcohol/Drug Problem Acknowledgement (ACK)	6	59	100
Alcohol/Drug Problem Proneness (PRO)	20	58	100
Immaturity Scale (IMM)	18	57	100
Anxiety (A)	33	76	100
Repression (R)	11	44	100
Depression Subscales (Harris-Lingoes)			
Subjective Depression (D1)	18	72	100
Psychomotor Retardation (D2)	7	61	100
Physical Malfunctioning (D3)	4	55	100
Mental Dullness (D4)	6	60	100
Brooding (D5)	8	76	100
Hysteria Subscales (Harris-Lingoes)			
Denial of Social Anxiety (Hy1)	1	38	100
Need for Affection (Hy2)	1	33	100
Lassitude-Malaise (Hy3)	9	70	100
Somatic Complaints (Hy4)	10	71	94
Inhibition of Aggression (Hy5)	2	44	100
Psychopathic Deviate Subscales (Harris-Lingoes)			
Familial Discord (Pd1)	3	48	100
Authority Problems (Pd2)	2	41	100
Social Imperturbability (Pd3)	0	30	100
Social Alienation (Pd4)	10	74	100
Self-Alienation (Pd5)	10	73	100
Paranoia Subscales (Harris-Lingoes)			
Persecutory Ideas (Pa1)	12	78	100
Poignancy (Pa2)	6	67	100
Naivete (Pa3)	1	34	100

Schizophrenia Subscales (Harris-Lingoes)

Social Alienation (Sc1)	11	65	100
Emotional Alienation (Sc2)	4	59	100
Lack of Ego Mastery, Cognitive (Sc3)	8	73	100
Lack of Ego Mastery, Conative (Sc4)	9	69	100
Lack of Ego Mastery, Defective Inhibition (Sc5)	9	77	100
Bizarre Sensory Experiences (Sc6)	11	68	95

Hypomania Subscales (Harris-Lingoes)

Amorality (Ma1)	2	45	100
Psychomotor Acceleration (Ma2)	8	57	100
Imperturbability (Ma3)	2	43	100
Ego Inflation (Ma4)	7	64	100

Social Introversion Subscales (Ben-Porath, Hostetler, Butcher, & Graham)

Shyness / Self-Consciousness (Si1)	11	65	100
Social Avoidance (Si2)	2	47	100
Alienation--Self and Others (Si3)	15	72	100

Uniform T scores are used for Hs, D, Hy, Pd, Pa, Pt, Sc, Ma, and the Content Scales; all other
MMPI-A scales use linear T scores.

OMITTED ITEMS

The following items were omitted by the client. It may be helpful to discuss these item omissions with this individual to determine the reason for non-compliance with test instructions.

172. I have had no difficulty in keeping my balance in walking.

End of Report

SUGGESTED ITEMS FOR FOLLOW-UP

ALCOHOL/DRUG PROBLEMS

144. I have a problem with alcohol or drugs. (T)

467. I enjoy using marijuana. (T)

SUICIDAL BEHAVIORS

177. I sometimes think about killing myself. (T)

FAMILY PROBLEMS

366. I have gotten many beatings. (T)

460. I have never run away from home. (F)

CASE 13
"MICHELLE"

A YOUNGSTER EXHIBITING
SEVERE PSYCHOTIC SYMPTOMS

BACKGROUND

Michelle is a 15–year–old, Caucasian female who was admitted to a secure residential setting as a transfer from a psychiatric hospital. She had been admitted to the hospital following an incident in which she locked herself in a locker at a day-treatment program. It was reported that she was experiencing command auditory hallucinations. While being transported to the hospital, Michelle set a fire in the police cruiser.

Michelle is the first of three children. She has a 12–year–old sister and a nine–year–old brother. There is a history of school and behavioral problems since the age of 13. She has been described as skipping school, being defiant, verbally aggressive, physically threatening and aggressive, and as bringing knives to school. There is no known history of drug or alcohol abuse or mental illness in her family.

Michelle was first treated by a psychologist at age 13 following an overdose with pills after a relationship with a boyfriend ended. Her mother was dissatisfied with her progress and transferred her to the care of a psychiatrist who treated her with psychotherapy and anxiolitic medication.

While under the care of the psychologist, she was administered the MMPI–A and the Draw A Person, and her mother completed the Conner's Parent Rating Scale. The MMPI–A was valid and reflected significant depression, possible suicidal tendencies, pervasive mistrust of others, and tendencies for oppositional and acting-out behavior. The DAP suggested mistrust of males and anxiety. The resultant diagnoses were Conduct Disorder, Solitary Aggressive Type; Depressive Disorder, NOS; and paranoid personality features.

When admitted to the psychiatric hospital, Michelle was seen as extremely combative and was reported to have set a fire in the seclusion room. She continued to experience auditory hallucinations and was prescribed Trilafon. The discharge diagnosis was that of Psychotic Disorder, NOS; R/O PTSD with dissociative features, Conduct Disorder, R/O Eating disorder, NOS, Probable Developmental Disorders and R/O developing Borderline Personality Disorder.

Upon admission to the intensive-care residential center, following her four–day hospitalization, Michelle was seen as exhibiting some mild loosening of associations as well as some confusion and possible thought blockage. Her affect was flattened and inappropriate to her mood which she related to be very depressed. It was also observed that she would laugh inappropriately at emotionally painful topics. Michelle denied current auditory hallucinations, stating that after being started on the Trilafon, the voices disappeared. She was not currently delusional and no formal paranoid ideation was elicited. She was fully oriented with no recall impairment. Insight and judgment were limited and below age expectations.

The Bender Visual Motor Gestalt, the Rorschach, and the Thematic Apperception Test were administered and the MMPI–A was readministered. The Bender record was scored using the Koppitz system and yielded no scoreable errors. The TAT was found to indicate significant themes of depression. Interpersonal relationships were portrayed as being distant and non-rewarding. The record was also suggestive of sexual preoccupation. The overall tone of the record was that of mistrust, loss, and separation. The Rorschach was notable for markedly unusual content. Youth with similar protocols are generally seen as exhibiting a thought disorder with idiosyncratic thinking. The record suggested a strong likelihood for paranoid ideation as well as poor emotional control. Predominate depression was suggested as well as considerable conflict with males. Interpersonally, she is likely to have difficulty with empathy, and may be seen as oppositional with difficulty conforming to the expectations of others.

MMPI–A INTERPRETATION
Profile Validity

Michelle's scores on the MMPI–A validity scales indicate that she, in all likelihood, produced a valid MMPI–A profile. She responded to all the test items and provided a consistent and coherent set of responses. Her score on VRIN indicates no tendency toward random responding, and her score on TRIN indicates only a minimal tendency toward inconsistent "True" responding. She produced an elevated score on F and its subscale F_1, and a much lower score on F_2.

The elevation on F indicates an unusual pattern of responding when compared to

the MMPI–A normative sample. Of the three possible causes for such a pattern, random responding, severe psychological problems, and over–reporting of symptoms, random responding can be ruled out on the basis of VRIN. We know from the background information that Michelle was experiencing very severe symptomatology, including auditory hallucinations, shortly before completing the MMPI–A. Her elevation on F can be attributed to these symptoms and, therefore, likely does not reflect over–reporting of symptoms. The discrepancy between F_1 and F_2 may also be explained in terms of Michelle's clinical presentation. Because most of the MMPI–A items describing psychotic symptoms are included in the clinical scales, they appear in the first half of the MMPI–A booklet. Therefore, an adolescent who is experiencing and reporting such symptoms is likely to score higher on F_1 than on F_2.

Finally, Michelle's scores on L and K, although slightly below normal, are not submerged to a point that would suggest that Michelle is overwhelmed by her symptoms. This too indicates a lesser likelihood of over–reporting of problems.

Overall, Michelle produced a valid MMPI–A profile. She responded to the test items in a relevant and consistent manner. She produced a relatively large number of unusual responses, which is consistent with her clinical presentation including severe psychological problems. Her scores on the MMPI–A clinical, content, and supplementary scales should produce a valid representation of her current functioning.

Current Level of Adjustment

Michelle's MMPI–A profile portrays a picture of chronic maladjustment characterized by severe behavioral discontrol and current psychotic symptomatology. It also indicates that her current level of distress is less severe than would be expected on the basis of her present difficulties and functioning. This interpretation is indicated by Michelle's pattern of scores on the test. Her elevations on Scale 4 and Adolescent Conduct Problems

(A–con) are equal to her elevations on Scale 6 and Scale 8 on the clinical profile and Adolescent Bizarre Mentation (A–biz) on the content scale profile. Both sets of scores are higher than her clinical scale elevations on Scale 2 and Scale 7 and content scale scores on Adolescent Anxiety (A–anx) and Adolescent Depression (A–dep). Also, Michelle's scores on L and K are not very low, as would be expected if she were feeling very distressed and overwhelmed by her current difficulties.

Thus, Michelle is currently experiencing severe psychological problems manifested by extreme acting-out tendencies and very unusual and, likely, psychotic symptoms. However, she is not feeling as anxious and overwhelmed by this situation as would be expected based on the severity of her problems.

Symptoms and Traits

Michelle produced highly elevated scores on clinical scales 4, 6, and 8. Her elevation on Scale 4 indicates that Michelle likely has a very strong tendency toward acting-out behavior, that she tends to be aggressive toward others and likely has significant adjustment problems in school, that she tends to be rebellious and, possibly, openly hostile toward authority figures, that she is impulsive and has difficulties delaying gratification, that she likely has severe conflict with members of her family, that she is prone to risk–taking and sensation–seeking behavior, that she may engage in substance abuse, and that she may experience relatively little emotional distress.

Her elevated score on Scale 6 indicates that Michelle tends to experience a considerable amount of anger, resentment, and hostility toward others, that she tends to project blame for her difficulties onto others, that she is suspicious of other people's intentions toward her, that she may experience persecutory delusions, and that she tends to be hypersensitive to perceived criticism by others.

Michelle's highly elevated score on Scale 8 indicates that she may presently be con-fused and disorganized, that she may be experiencing psychotic symptoms including delusions and hallucinations, that she may have poor reality testing at this time, and that she probably feels alienated from others and unable to form close relationships.

Michelle also produced an unusually high score on clinical Scale 5. Although this scale has very limited utility in clinical interpretation, Michelle's particularly elevated score on this scale indicates that she may reject traditional feminine interests and may have some confusion about her sexual identity.

Michelle produced secondary elevations on clinical scales 1, 2, and 7, indicating that she reports experiencing some unpleasant affect at this time, coupled with some physical complaints. She may report feeling somewhat depressed and anxious and is likely to complain of some vague somatic problems. Her severe acting-out tendencies coupled with complaints of depression indicate the possibility of some suicide risk. Examination of the list of Suggested Items for Follow–up indicates that Michelle does, indeed, report some suicidal ideation at this time.

Michelle's scores on the MMPI–A Content Scales indicate interpretations that are similar to those suggested by the clinical scales. Her elevation on Adolescent Conduct Problems (A–con) indicates that Michelle acknowledges engaging in severe acting-out behaviors and suggests that she has very poor impulse control and that she holds socially deviant beliefs and attitudes. Her level of elevation on this scale indicates that Michelle's conduct problems are very severe, and that she is not reluctant to acknowledge her socially deviant behaviors and attitudes. Thus, Michelle is likely to exhibit little or no remorse for her acting-out behaviors and the difficulties they may cause her and others.

Her elevated score on the Adolescent School Problems (A–sch) scale indicates that Michelle's acting-out tendencies are likely to create substantial difficulties for her at school. She is likely to have severe disciplinary problems as well as academic difficulties. Her elevation on Adolescent Family Problems (A–fam) indicates that Michelle reports substantial problems in her relationships with members of her family, whom she may tend to blame for her problems. Her elevated score on this scale also indicates that Michelle likely views her family as a source of strife and conflict, rather than support.

Michelle's highly elevated score on Adolescent Bizarre Mentation (A–biz) indicates that she reports a large number of very unusual experiences including delusions and hallucinations. Because (as discussed later) she also likely engages in drug abuse, the possibility exists that some of her bizarre experiences may be drug induced. Regardless of their cause, Michelle's highly elevated score on this scale indicates that her problems in this area are severe and in need of immediate attention.

Michelle also produced an elevated score on the Adolescent Cynicism (A–cyn) scale, indicating that she tends to be very mistrustful of the motives of others, that she believes that people tend to look out only for their own interests, and that she likely is suspicious of anyone who attempts to be friendly toward her. Her elevation on Adolescent Alienation (A–aln) is consistent with this tendency and indicates that Michelle feels emotionally distant from others and unable to form warm emotional ties. She views others as a source of threat, rather than comfort or assistance.

Michelle also produced an elevated score on Adolescent Depression (A–dep), indicating that she reports feeling somewhat dysphoric at this time. She may indicate having a low drive and may experience suicidal ideation. Michelle's score on Adolescent Anxiety (A–anx) indicates that she is experiencing some subjective symptoms of anxiety and discomfort at this time. However, as already discussed, her level of anxiety and distress is considerably lower than would be expected in light of the severity of her current difficulties. Her elevated score on Adolescent Health Concerns (A–hea) indicates that Michelle complains of a number of physical health problems at this time.

Finally, Michelle's highest score on the content scales is on the Adolescent Negative Treatment Indicators (A–trt) scale. In fact, Michelle obtained nearly the highest score possible on this scale. This indicates that she tends to be very mistrustful of mental health professionals, that she may not believe that she needs professional assistance at this time, and that she presently has a very low motivation for treatment. Obviously, all these characteristics have serious implications for her treatment. These will be discussed below under treatment recommendations.

Overall, Michelle's MMPI–A profile indicates that she likely has severe behavioral control and acting-out problems, that she tends to be rebellious toward figures of authority, that she likely has disciplinary and academic problems in school as well as serious conflicts with members of her family. She tends to be resentful and angry and is inclined to blame others for her difficulties. Michelle is very suspicious and mistrustful of others and she may presently be experiencing persecutory delusions. In addition, she may at this time be confused and disorganized and she may be experiencing psychotic symptoms including delusions and hallucinations. She may have poor reality testing and may feel alienated from others. Michelle may also be experiencing difficulties in the area of sexual identity.

Additional indications in Michelle's MMPI–A profile are that she is experiencing some depression at this time. In light of her depression and impulsive tendencies, she may be at risk for a suicide attempt or gesture. She may also be concerned about physical health matters.

Diagnostic Suggestions

Michelle's MMPI–A profile raises concerns about several possible diagnoses that need to be examined further. Her scores on Scales 6, 8, and A–biz indicate the likelihood of psychotic symptomatology. The possibility of an early stage of schizophrenia needs to be explored. The likelihood that Michelle's psychotic symptoms may be manifestations of the early stages of a severe borderline personality disorder needs also to be explored. This possibility is also indicated by Michelle's behavioral discontrol, emotional lability, and identity confusion that are reflected in her MMPI–A profile. The possibility that at least some of the very bizarre symptoms that Michelle describes may be induced by drug use also needs to be explored.

Michelle's MMPI–A profile is strongly suggestive of a conduct disorder characterized by aggression, destructiveness, deceitfulness, and serious rule violations. Her level of elevation on MMPI–A conduct disorder indicators suggests that her disorder is likely to be classified as severe. The relative absence of anxiety in Michelle's MMPI–A profile points toward a psychopathic personality structure underlying her conduct disorder.

The possibility of a depressive disorder also warrants further examination. Michelle produced an elevated score on A–dep indicating the presence of dysphoric affect and other symptoms of depression. She also endorsed an item reflective of suicidal ideation. All of these indicate the need to evaluate further whether Michelle meets diagnostic criteria for a depressive disorder.

Examination of the Suggested Items for Follow–up indicates that Michelle endorsed an item reflective of bulimic tendencies. Although an adolescent's response to a single item is in no way sufficient to indicate the presence, or even the likelihood, of a problem, this response can be viewed as a "red flag" in need of follow–up and further evaluation.

Michelle's scores on the MMPI–A supplementary scales also point to some serious concerns. She produced a highly elevated score on the Revised MacAndrew (MAC–R) scale indicating that she is at very high risk for having an alcohol and/or drug problem. Consistent with other MMPI–A indicators, this score suggests that Michelle has very strong tendencies toward risk-taking and

sensation-seeking and that the abuse of alcohol and drugs may be one way in which she acts upon these tendencies. Her highly elevated score on the Alcohol/Drug Problem Proneness (PRO) scale bolsters the concerns raised by her score on MAC–R and adds the strong possibility that Michelle tends to be highly influenced by negative peers who may also reinforce her proclivity toward alcohol and drug use. Finally, Michelle's elevated score on the Alcohol/Drug Problem Acknowledgment (ACK) scale indicates that she readily acknowledges her problems in this area and, in fact, may admit them in an openly defiant manner. Examination of the Suggested Items for Follow–up indicates that Michelle acknowledges the use of both alcohol and marijuana.

Treatment Recommendations

Michelle's MMPI–A profile indicates that she likely is experiencing psychotic symptoms at this time. A referral for a psychiatric evaluation to determine her need for antipsychotic medication is therefore suggested. Examination of, and attention to, Michelle's risk for suicidal behavior is indicated by her depressed mood, endorsement of an item reflective of suicidal ideation, by her emotional lability, and by her tendencies toward very impulsive behavior. As just indicated under diagnostic suggestions, further evaluation of the possibility that Michelle may have an eating disorder is indicated.

Once her psychotic symptoms are controlled, it is very likely that Michelle will continue to exhibit severe behavioral control problems. Development of a highly structured contingency–based behavioral management program is recommended. An evaluation for substance-use problems is also indicated.

The prospects for Michelle's treatment are, unfortunately, limited. Her highly elevated score on A–trt indicates that she does not trust mental-health professionals, likely has severe difficulties opening up and sharing her problems with others, has very low motivation for treatment, and may not believe that there is anything wrong with her that requires treatment. Further, in spite of the severe nature of her current difficulties, Michelle is experiencing relatively little anxiety and therefore is unlikely to be highly motivated for treatment. Nevertheless, it is recommended that an effort be made to engage Michelle in individual therapy in an attempt to provide her with a positive interpersonal experience.

OUTCOME

Michelle's diagnoses following this evaluation were Psychotic Disorder, NOS; Dysthymic Disorder; a developing personality disorder with Borderline features; Conduct Disorder, Adolescent–Onset Type, Severe; and Polysubstance abuse. The potential for a schizophrenic disorder was also suggested.

Michelle was maintained in a structured clinical setting, although her initial placement was only to be two weeks. Follow–up meetings with the referral agencies resulted in approval for continued treatment with 30-day reviews. She was continued on antipsychotic medication. She was seen first in relationship-oriented therapy with the goal of increasing her ability to form a therapeutic bond as well as strengthening reality ties. In addition, cognitive–behav-

ioral therapy focussing on impulse control, self-image, depression, and anger management was introduced after the initial stages of psychotherapy. Michelle received art therapy with a focus on identification, expression and control of emotions. She was enrolled in a girls' therapy group that focussed on interpersonal relations, emotional management, social skills, and trauma-related issues. Michelle was referred to substance-abuse counseling and an eating disorder consultant was engaged to assist the treatment team.

Michelle has shown a somewhat favorable response to treatment with gains in reality testing and no indications of perceptual abnormalities. Her affect is now stable and appropriate. She is able to engage in conflict resolution with her mother. She continues to have severe behavioral problems. Although she has not assaulted anyone or required restraint, she remains defiant of structure and tends to link with other youth who have conduct problems. She has begun to participate in a structured interpersonal skills group on the unit as well as recreational therapy. The current goal is placement in a treatment foster home with day placement in a partial hospitalization program.

MMPI-A*

Extended Score Report

ID Number 13

Michelle

Female

Age 15

4/11/94

MMPI-A BASIC SCALES PROFILE

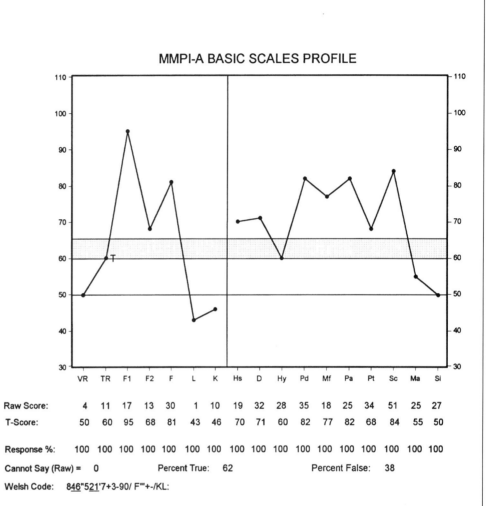

	VR	TR	F1	F2	F	L	K	Hs	D	Hy	Pd	Mf	Pa	Pt	Sc	Ma	Si
Raw Score:	4	11	17	13	30	1	10	19	32	28	35	18	25	34	51	25	27
T-Score:	50	60	95	68	81	43	46	70	71	60	82	77	82	68	84	55	50
Response %:	100	100	100	100	100	100	100	100	100	100	100	100	100	100	100	100	100

Cannot Say (Raw) =   0   Percent True: 62   Percent False: 38

Welsh Code: 846"521'7+3-90/ F'''+-/KL:

CASE 13
"MICHELLE"

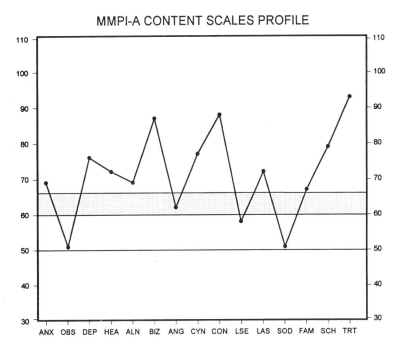

MMPI-A CONTENT SCALES PROFILE

	ANX	OBS	DEP	HEA	ALN	BIZ	ANG	CYN	CON	LSE	LAS	SOD	FAM	SCH	TRT
Raw Score:	16	9	21	21	12	15	12	21	20	9	11	8	21	14	23
T-Score:	69	51	76	72	69	87	62	77	88	58	72	51	67	79	93
Response %:	100	100	100	100	100	100	100	100	100	100	100	100	100	100	100

SUPPLEMENTARY SCORE REPORT

	Raw Score	T Score	Resp %
MacAndrew Alcoholism-Revised (MAC-R)	35	87	100
Alcohol/Drug Problem Acknowledgement (ACK)	10	77	100
Alcohol/Drug Problem Proneness (PRO)	29	79	100
Immaturity Scale (IMM)	28	76	100
Anxiety (A)	29	66	100
Repression (R)	10	40	100
Depression Subscales (Harris-Lingoes)			
Subjective Depression (D1)	19	70	100
Psychomotor Retardation (D2)	6	57	100
Physical Malfunctioning (D3)	6	64	100
Mental Dullness (D4)	8	66	100
Brooding (D5)	7	65	100
Hysteria Subscales (Harris-Lingoes)			
Denial of Social Anxiety (Hy1)	4	54	100
Need for Affection (Hy2)	3	42	100
Lassitude-Malaise (Hy3)	10	69	100
Somatic Complaints (Hy4)	9	63	100
Inhibition of Aggression (Hy5)	1	35	100
Psychopathic Deviate Subscales (Harris-Lingoes)			
Familial Discord (Pd1)	5	56	100
Authority Problems (Pd2)	7	79	100
Social Imperturbability (Pd3)	4	55	100
Social Alienation (Pd4)	9	66	100
Self-Alienation (Pd5)	10	71	100
Paranoia Subscales (Harris-Lingoes)			
Persecutory Ideas (Pa1)	14	87	100
Poignancy (Pa2)	6	62	100
Naivete (Pa3)	1	36	100

Schizophrenia Subscales (Harris-Lingoes)

Social Alienation (Sc1)	13	70	100
Emotional Alienation (Sc2)	5	65	100
Lack of Ego Mastery, Cognitive (Sc3)	7	67	100
Lack of Ego Mastery, Conative (Sc4)	9	67	100
Lack of Ego Mastery, Defective Inhibition (Sc5)	8	68	100
Bizarre Sensory Experiences (Sc6)	16	81	100

Hypomania Subscales (Harris-Lingoes)

Amorality (Ma1)	4	63	100
Psychomotor Acceleration (Ma2)	5	39	100
Imperturbability (Ma3)	3	50	100
Ego Inflation (Ma4)	6	58	100

Social Introversion Subscales (Ben-Porath, Hostetler, Butcher, & Graham)

Shyness / Self-Consciousness (Si1)	1	34	100
Social Avoidance (Si2)	2	51	100
Alienation--Self and Others (Si3)	15	68	100

Uniform T scores are used for Hs, D, Hy, Pd, Pa, Pt, Sc, Ma, and the Content Scales; all other MMPI-A scales use linear T scores.

End of Report

SUGGESTED ITEMS FOR FOLLOW-UP

ALCOHOL/DRUG PROBLEMS

161. I have had periods in which I carried on activities without knowing later what I had been doing. (T)

247. I have used alcohol excessively. (T)

431. Talking over problems and worries with someone is often more helpful than taking drugs or medicines. (F)

458. I sometimes get into fights when drinking. (T)

467. I enjoy using marijuana. (T)

EATING DISORDER SYMPTOMS

108. Sometimes I make myself throw up after eating so I won't gain weight. (T)

SUICIDAL BEHAVIORS

283. Most of the time I wish I were dead. (T)

FAMILY PROBLEMS

440. I have spent nights away from home when my parents did not know where I was. (T)

460. I have never run away from home. (F)

CASE 14
"NED"

A JUVENILE BINDOVER EVALUATION WITH QUESTIONS REGARDING THE ORIGIN OF SEVERE IMPULSE CONTROL PROBLEMS

BACKGROUND

Ned is a 16-year-old, Caucasian male referred by his attorney for a forensic psychological evaluation. The purpose of the evaluation was to determine potential for rehabilitation as part of a bindover hearing held in juvenile court.

Ned was charged with Aggravated Murder. It was alleged that, as part of a gang initiation rite, he walked up to a young boy and shot him at close range. The victim died immediately and, when apprehended by the police, Ned confessed to his involvement in the shooting.

Ned was seen six times in a juvenile detention center. He was interviewed and the following diagnostic psychological tests were administered: the MMPI–A/taped administration; the Thematic Apperception Test (TAT); the Rorschach; the Ammons Quick Test of Intelligence; the Bender Visual Motor Gestalt Test; the Draw A Person (DAP); and the Kinetic Family Drawing. In addition, his mother and step-father were interviewed.

Ned is the only child born of the marriage of his parents. His mother reported no birth complication or trauma with the delivery, but Ned was two weeks overdue. He met major developmental milestones appropriately. He

walked at nine months of age. Ned did not have any serious illnesses or injuries from infancy to the time of evaluation.

The mother alleged that Ned's father physically abused her. He was usually unemployed and he was further described as having a short temper. The mother denied that Ned witnessed or experienced any of the abuse. However, Ned reported that his father "pulled guns" on his mother and that his father gave her a face fracture. Ned denied any sexual abuse. There is a notation of one investigation by Children's Services but both the youth and the parents deny that any abuse actually took place.

Ned's parents divorced one year after his birth. The divorce was uncontested and his mother later remarried. Ned was four years old at the time of this union. Two other children were born from this marriage and Ned resided with his mother, step-father, and half-siblings at the time of the alleged offense.

The biological father was not a consistent figure in Ned's life. He stated that his father would give him cigarettes and other minor items but was not there for emotional support. Ned reported that his father "used to drink alcohol, do acid and dope." He described his father as "a walking time bomb." The father is reported to have belonged to two motorcycle gangs. He has been incarcerated periodically for various felonies. Ned stated that he has nine step–siblings, ranging from 13 to 30 years of age, as a result of his father's eight marriages.

Ned started preschool at three years of age. During the first grade his teachers noticed signs of hyperactivity. He was unable to concentrate. He was retained in the first, third, and ninth grades. He was diagnosed as evidencing Attention Deficit Hyperactivity Disorder. Ned was prescribed Ritalin in elementary school. He reported that he took Ritalin from the second grade through the fourth or fifth grade. Ritalin was, however, discontinued after the sixth grade by his parents after Ned continued to complain of a side-effect of sleeplessness. Mental health and medical records indicate an inconsistent pattern of Ritalin usage before discontinuation.

According to educational records, Ned was identified as having a Specific Learning Disability and a Language Disorder. He began to exhibit negative behaviors in Middle School. He was suspended for fighting twice. Records indicate a history of suspensions, as well, for insubordination and classroom disruption. Ned was placed in high school at the age of 16 and was in his freshman year at the time of the alleged offense. He was in Specific Learning Disability classes and felt like "I was in the stupid classes."

The parents reported that in the summer before Ned started high school they noticed he had a fascination with gangs. He began wearing gang–related paraphernalia such as head bands. He also talked frequently of gangs. Ned stated that he has been involved in a gang since before high school. There is no history, however, of juvenile court involvement. Ned's parents denied significant home behavioral problems. They claimed that the night of the alleged offense was the first night in which he stayed out overnight without permission and that they went looking for him that night. They denied that he had any history of fire-set-

ting or cruelty to animals. They stated that he was not disobedient at home and did not have a problem with theft.

Ned had been employed in fast-food restaurants. These jobs exceeded his capabilities and he was terminated from them. Ned wrestled at a recreational facility for three years and had won a trophy each year. He participated in roller skating frequently on Fridays until two a.m.

Ned admitted to smoking marijuana on the weekends in addition to consuming alcohol since 14 years of age. He claimed to be sexually active. He stated that he first became involved in sexual play when he was nine years old. He claimed that his sexual experiences had occurred with girls ranging from "my age" to an encounter with a 17–year–old when he was 12.

Ned was evaluated in a series of two-hour sessions that consisted of interviews and test administrations. The need for repeated evaluations resulted from his severe attentional difficulties.

In the evaluations, Ned was dressed in clothing issued by the detention home. His hygiene was often quite poor, owing, he stated, to his being placed in administrative isolation and being unable to shave and shower on a daily basis. There was noticeable acne on his face, which he stated had worsened since his confinement. At times, there was a noticeable body odor about him. His gait and posture were non-remarkable. There were no indications of gross or fine motor dysfunction. He was left–hand dominant. His level of psychomotor activity was significantly elevated throughout all the sessions. He would require frequent refocussing and redirection to complete tasks. He would often require redirection to return to the topic of conversation. He was highly distractible to outside stimuli, to the extent that the shades on the office window would need to be drawn in order for him to focus attention. His speech was often pressured and rapid. There were flights of ideas noted, that is, his conversation would often move quickly from one topic to another without the first concepts often being finished.

Ned was not tangential and did not evidence loosening of associations or other indications of a disorder in the form of his thinking. His eye contact was direct. His manner of interaction was cooperative, but markedly socially immature. He attempted all tasks requested of him. His approach to problem-solving was a nonsystematic, trial and error manner. He presented interpersonally as a socially immature youth who attempted to be far more sophisticated than his social skills would indicate.

Ned presented a mildly labile affect to a stated anxious and depressed mood. He denied experiencing, and there were no indications of, perceptual abnormalities such as visual, auditory, tactile, olfactory, or gustatory hallucinations. He was seen to evidence variations in his mood from being depressed to elevated and expansive at times. He expressed the belief that persons wanted to harm him and stated that he had death threats against him. No specific, organized paranoid ideation or systems were elicited, however. There were no current indications of compulsions or obsessions. As noted, he acknowledged considerable depression and stated that he felt considerable guilt over his alleged actions. He reported fitful and poor sleep with frequent nightmares. His appetite was undisturbed. He denied thoughts of suicide or harming others. He was oriented to time, place, and person. His long-term, short-term and immediate-recall functions appeared to be clinically intact. His insight and judgment appeared to be markedly below age expectations.

On the Ammons Quick Test, a verbal perceptual measure of general intelligence, Ned was found to function in the low average range of general intellectual functioning. This finding is commensurate with previous intellectual evaluations. Ned's Bender record was scored using the Koppitz system. Analysis found errors of partial rotation, angulation, distortion, and expansiveness. The record was found to be similar to those associated with certain types of neuropsychological dysfunction and, in particular, learning disabilities. Qualitatively, the record suggests tendencies for impulsiveness. The projective drawings indicate that he has a markedly poor self-image, immature social skills, and limited problem-solving capacities. He appears to have considerable dependency needs and a fairly immature view of interpersonal relationships. On the Thematic Apperception Test considerably immature social skills are also seen in his portrayals. He also expressed marked dependency needs and conflicts over meeting them. Persons with such patterns are often easily frustrated interpersonally because they lack the wherewithal to meet their needs and may be quite vulnerable to manipulation by others more socially adroit than they. Ned appears to have an external locus of control, that is, he places little faith in his own abilities or efforts to modify events in his life and tends to depend on outside influences. The protocol indicates pervasive feelings of depression and anxiety which may be overwhelming, although he typically will attempt to repress and deny such feelings. Ned appears to have strong feelings of anger and may be impulsive in his acting out of emotional conflicts. Lastly, the record suggests a markedly poor self-image.

Ned's Rorschach record was found to be similar to those associated with youth who have significant emotional problems. His manner of perception and pattern of responses are similar to those associated with persons who experience strong feelings of depression and have difficulty with emotional control. Persons with similar records have exhibited suicidal ideation and/or suicidal behavior. Conflicts with persons perceived as being in authority are often associated with similar records. He appears to be neglectful of details in his environment and may be quite impulsive. His problem-solving skills are likely quite deficient. Persons with similar records tend to have difficulty trusting others and may evidence a guarded interpersonal interactional pattern. Considerable preoccupation with somatic functioning is also suggested.

MMPI-A INTERPRETATION
Profile Validity

Ned produced a valid MMPI-A profile. He responded to all the test items and produced a consistent and coherent set of responses. He had a slightly elevated score on TRIN indicating an inconsequential tendency toward inconsistent "True" responding. His scores on F and its subscales are somewhat elevated, indicating that Ned reports experiencing a limited set of psychological problems at this time. His scores on L and K are within normal limits and unremarkable. Overall, Ned's MMPI-A profile should yield an accurate picture of his current psychological functioning.

Current Level of Adjustment

Ned's scores on the MMPI-A indicate that he is experiencing some psychological distress at this time. He produced elevated scores on six of the eight clinical scales, with one score, on Scale 9, being extremely elevated. Ned also produced several elevated scores on the content scales, including a highly elevated score on Adolescent Anxiety (A-anx), indicating that he is experiencing considerable psychological distress at this time. Ned's MMPI-A profile also indicates a tendency toward chronic maladjustment problems that are manifested in poor impulse-control and acting-out behaviors.

Symptoms and Traits

Ned produced an extremely elevated score on Scale 9. His score on this scale indicates that Ned tends to be very impulsive and restless. He is likely to be inclined toward irresponsible acting-out behavior. Ned's score on this scale suggests further that he may have a very unrealistically positive self-view, and that he is prone to grandiose thinking. Ned is likely to be emotionally labile, possibly experiencing extreme swings between a euphoric and dysphoric mood. He may experience flight of ideas, and his speech may appear to be pressured. He may have substantial difficulties maintaining his attention and concentration. He may present initially as being very outgoing

and friendly. He may be viewed as being energetic and talkative. However, he is likely to be very self-focussed.

Ned also produced a highly elevated score on Scale 1. His score on this scale indicates that Ned experiences considerable somatic and bodily concerns that may be vague in nature. His concerns are likely to focus on a number of different bodily systems. He may be prone to responding to stress by developing physical health problems and concerns. He is likely to be viewed by others as self-centered and cynical. Ned also produced an elevated score on Scale 3. This reinforces the impression that he is prone to developing physical problems in response to stressful situations. Examination of the relevant subscales also indicates that much of Ned's elevation on this scale stems from physical health concerns.

Ned's elevated score on Scale 6 is not uncommon in individuals charged with serious crimes who complete the MMPI-A in the context of a forensic evaluation. Examination of his scores on the relevant subscales indicates that Ned's elevation on this scale stems from persecutory beliefs and a hypersensitivity to criticism. Examination of the nature of Ned's persecutory beliefs may reveal that he fears retribution from family members or friends of his victim.

Ned produced a moderately elevated score on Scale 7, indicating that he is experiencing some anxiety and distress at this time. He may also be prone to obsessive rumination and may be experiencing feelings of shame and guilt. Ned also may have a negative-self view.

Examination of Ned's scores on the relevant subscales indicates that much of his elevation on Scale 8 is related to reports of Bizarre Sensory Experiences. These may include bizarre bodily sensations as well as unusual perceptual experiences. His subscales also indicate that Ned may be feeling that he is losing control over his thoughts and impulses. Ned produced a markedly low score on Scale 0, indicating that he presents as being very outgoing and extraverted and very comfortable in social situations.

His scores on the MMPI–A content scales confirm that Ned is very preoccupied with current physical health concerns. He produced a highly elevated score on Adolescent Health Concerns (A–hea), indicating a generalized preoccupation with his health as well as a reporting of numerous specific worries about his health. Ned's elevated score on Adolescent Anxiety (A–anx) indicates that he reports feeling substantial emotional distress at this time. He is likely very nervous and tense and may feel as though he is losing control over his mind. Ned also produced an elevated score on Adolescent Obsessiveness (A–obs) reinforcing indications in his clinical scales that he is prone to obsessive rumination, that he tends to become overly worrisome and preoccupied, and likely has difficulties making decisions.

Ned's elevated score on Adolescent Anger (A–ang) indicates that he acknowledges having anger management problems. He likely tends to be irritable and may over–respond to seemingly minor provocation. Ned is likely to be viewed as aggressive and he may become involved in physical altercations. His score on Adolescent Cynicism (A–cyn) indicates that Ned holds misanthropic beliefs about others. He views other people with suspicion, particularly when they are being nice to him for no apparent reason. He is mistrustful of others and disinclined to form strong relationships. His low score on Adolescent Social Discomfort (A–sod) indicates that in spite of Ned's misanthropic tendencies, he is comfortable in social situations and may create the facade of openness and friendliness.

Ned's score on Adolescent Conduct Problems (A–con) indicates that he acknowledges engaging in antisocial behavior and holding antisocial attitudes. He may act out aggressively toward others and generally disrespects the rights and feelings of others. His highly elevated score on Adolescent School Problems (A–sch) suggests that Ned's acting-out tendencies may be particularly pronounced in school, and that as a result he may have significant disciplinary and academic problems.

Ned's MMPI–A profile is also noteworthy for the low score he produced on Adolescent Low Aspirations (A–las). This score indicates that Ned has not given up on his future and that he continues to aspire to develop himself and achieve success. In light of his present legal situation, these aspirations may be somewhat unrealistic.

Overall, Ned's MMPI–A profile indicates a very strong tendency toward impulsive and irresponsible acting-out behavior, a high likelihood that he may be experiencing an excessive amount of energy manifested in pressured speech, flight of ideas, and, possibly, loose associations, a proclivity toward risk–taking and sensation–seeking, a likelihood that he has an overly–positive, perhaps grandiose, self-view, and the likelihood that he experiences difficulties in the areas of attention and concentration. Ned also tends to experience anger-control problems and he may be inclined toward aggressive interpersonal behavior. He is inclined toward extreme acting-out behavior and, as a result, may be experiencing substantial disciplinary and academic problems at school.

Ned's profile also indicates a strong preoccupation with somatic and bodily functions. He may be inclined toward developing physical symptoms in response to stress, and Ned may have some genuine physical problems that require medical attention. Ned's scores also indicate that he is experiencing a considerable amount of subjective anxiety at this time, that he tends toward obsessive rumination, and that he may be experiencing feelings of shame and guilt.

Ned's profile also indicates that he tends to be suspicious of others and that he has cynical interpersonal mistrust. Nevertheless, Ned is able to present as being very comfortable in social situations and he is likely to create a very favorable first impression on others.

Diagnostic Suggestions

Ned's MMPI–A profile presents some interesting issues for consideration in iden-

CASE 14
"NED"

tifying the appropriate diagnoses in his case. His highly elevated score on Scale 9 indicates the strong possibility of a manic episode which may be a manifestation of a bipolar disorder. To some extent, this score could also be reflective of a severe attention deficit disorder. However, the level of elevation on Scale 9 suggests the presence of symptoms that could not be accounted for completely by attentional deficits.

His elevation on Scale 8 and its subscales indicates the possibility that Ned may be experiencing psychotic symptoms. However, his score on the content scale Adolescent Bizarre Mentation (A–biz), although elevated, is not nearly as elevated as the subscale for Scale 8 called Bizarre Sensory Experiences. In addition, Ned has no known history of psychotic symptoms. This combination of indications points toward several possible interpretations of Ned's score on Scale 8.

It is possible that this score reflects psychotic features that may be accompanying a manic episode or a mood disorder. However, in light of his substantial elevation on Scale 1, the possibility of an organic basis for Ned's elevation on Scale 8 must be considered. Research with adults indicates that individuals with seizure disorders, closed head injuries, and other neurological conditions produce elevations on the subscale Bizarre Sensory Experiences. They also produce elevated scores on Scale 1. Thus, it is *possible* that some of Ned's physical and sensory complaints have an organic basis. This also *may* play a role in extreme mood swings and acting-out behaviors. Another possibility that should be weighed in considering Ned's scores on these scales is the potential effect of drugs. As discussed next, Ned's MMPI–A profile provides strong indications that he uses drugs, which may play a role in some of the unusual experiences he reports.

Other diagnostic possibilities raised by Ned's MMPI–A profile include a Conduct Disorder and a substance-use disorder. Examination of Ned's scores on the MMPI–A substance-use scales indicates

that he produced significantly elevated scores on all three scales. His elevated score on the Revised MacAndrew (MAC–R) scale indicates that Ned's tendency toward sensation–seeking and risk–taking behavior places him at substantial risk for developing a substance-use problem. His elevated score on the Alcohol/Drug Problems Proneness (PRO) scale reinforces this impression and indicates that involvement with negative peer groups may also play a role in making Ned vulnerable to developing a substance-use problem. Finally, his elevation on the Alcohol/Drug Problems Acknowledgment (ACK) scale indicates that Ned does in fact admit having problems in this area. Examination of his responses to the Suggested Items for Follow–up indicates that Ned acknowledges using both alcohol and marijuana.

Treatment Recommendations

Although a forensic evaluation such as the one that led to Ned's current testing with the MMPI–A may not call for specific treatment recommendations, suggestions for follow–up and the question of Ned's amenability to treatment are relevant.

A very important issue that requires follow–up is the nature and origin of Ned's unusual perceptual experiences and physical health complaints. The MMPI–A can only provide suggestive information regarding possible organic involvement in Ned's condition. The need for follow–up physical, neurological, and neuropsychological examination is suggested strongly by these data.

If the suggested evaluations identify organic conditions that may account for some of Ned's problems, then medical intervention would likely be indicated. Regardless of their origin, if follow–up examinations indicate the presence of psychotic symptoms, then a psychiatric examination for possible anti–psychotic medication may be indicated.

If organic causes are ruled out, and Ned's extreme acting-out behavior is viewed primarily as a function of a conduct disorder, then behavioral intervention may be indicated. In light of the circumstances of the evaluation, such intervention would most likely be provided in a juvenile correctional facility. Individual and group therapy designed to assist Ned in acquiring greater trust in others may also be indicated. Overall, the prognosis for treatment will depend to a large extent on the final formulation of the origin of Ned's problems.

OUTCOME

The psychologist's report contained recommendations for follow–up physical, neurological, and neuropsychological examinations. Diagnosis was deferred until the results of those evaluations were available.

CASE 14
"NED"

CASE 14
"NED"

MMPI-A*

Extended Score Report

ID Number 14

Ned

Male

Age 16

11/27/94

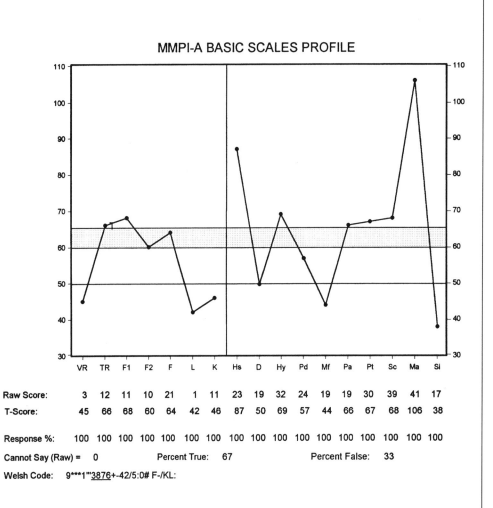

MMPI-A BASIC SCALES PROFILE

	VR	TR	F1	F2	F	L	K	Hs	D	Hy	Pd	Mf	Pa	Pt	Sc	Ma	Si
Raw Score:	3	12	11	10	21	1	11	23	19	32	24	19	19	30	39	41	17
T-Score:	45	66	68	60	64	42	46	87	50	69	57	44	66	67	68	106	38
Response %:	100	100	100	100	100	100	100	100	100	100	100	100	100	100	100	100	100

Cannot Say (Raw) = 0   Percent True: 67   Percent False: 33

Welsh Code: 9***1'''3876+-42/5:0# F-/KL:

CASE 14
"NED"

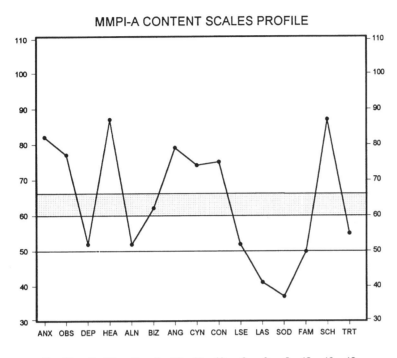

MMPI-A CONTENT SCALES PROFILE

	ANX	OBS	DEP	HEA	ALN	BIZ	ANG	CYN	CON	LSE	LAS	SOD	FAM	SCH	TRT
Raw Score:	19	14	9	25	7	8	15	20	18	6	3	2	12	16	12
T-Score:	82	77	52	87	52	62	79	74	75	52	41	37	50	87	55
Response %:	100	100	100	100	100	100	100	100	100	100	100	100	100	100	100

SUPPLEMENTARY SCORE REPORT

	Raw Score	T Score	Resp %
MacAndrew Alcoholism-Revised (MAC-R)	33	77	100
Alcohol/Drug Problem Acknowledgement (ACK)	10	75	100
Alcohol/Drug Problem Proneness (PRO)	26	71	100
Immaturity Scale (IMM)	23	65	100
Anxiety (A)	25	65	100
Repression (R)	5	31	100
Depression Subscales (Harris-Lingoes)			
Subjective Depression (D1)	12	58	100
Psychomotor Retardation (D2)	2	36	100
Physical Malfunctioning (D3)	6	68	100
Mental Dullness (D4)	6	60	100
Brooding (D5)	2	46	100
Hysteria Subscales (Harris-Lingoes)			
Denial of Social Anxiety (Hy1)	5	61	100
Need for Affection (Hy2)	5	50	100
Lassitude-Malaise (Hy3)	7	62	100
Somatic Complaints (Hy4)	14	85	100
Inhibition of Aggression (Hy5)	0	30	100
Psychopathic Deviate Subscales (Harris-Lingoes)			
Familial Discord (Pd1)	1	37	100
Authority Problems (Pd2)	5	60	100
Social Imperturbability (Pd3)	5	61	100
Social Alienation (Pd4)	7	60	100
Self-Alienation (Pd5)	7	61	100
Paranoia Subscales (Harris-Lingoes)			
Persecutory Ideas (Pa1)	10	71	100
Poignancy (Pa2)	6	67	100
Naivete (Pa3)	2	40	100

CASE 14
"NED"

Schizophrenia Subscales (Harris-Lingoes)

Social Alienation (Sc1)	7	53	100
Emotional Alienation (Sc2)	3	54	100
Lack of Ego Mastery, Cognitive (Sc3)	7	68	100
Lack of Ego Mastery, Conative (Sc4)	8	65	100
Lack of Ego Mastery, Defective Inhibition (Sc5)	6	62	100
Bizarre Sensory Experiences (Sc6)	15	80	100

Hypomania Subscales (Harris-Lingoes)

Amorality (Ma1)	6	73	100
Psychomotor Acceleration (Ma2)	11	71	100
Imperturbability (Ma3)	7	74	100
Ego Inflation (Ma4)	8	69	100

Social Introversion Subscales (Ben-Porath, Hostetler, Butcher, & Graham)

Shyness / Self-Consciousness (Si1)	0	30	100
Social Avoidance (Si2)	0	38	100
Alienation--Self and Others (Si3)	10	57	100

Uniform T scores are used for Hs, D, Hy, Pd, Pa, Pt, Sc, Ma, and the Content Scales; all other MMPI-A scales use linear T scores.

End of Report

SUGGESTED ITEMS FOR FOLLOW-UP

ALCOHOL/DRUG PROBLEMS

144. I have a problem with alcohol or drugs. (T)

161. I have had periods in which I carried on activities without knowing later what I had been doing. (T)

247. I have used alcohol excessively. (T)

342. I can express my true feelings only when I drink. (T)

458. I sometimes get into fights when drinking. (T)

467. I enjoy using marijuana. (T)

474. People often tell me I have a problem with drinking too much. (T)

FAMILY PROBLEMS

440. I have spent nights away from home when my parents did not know where I was. (T)

CASE 15

"OLIVER"

A YOUNGSTER EXPERIENCING A
MANIC EPISODE WITH PSYCHOTIC FEATURES

BACKGROUND

Oliver is a 14-year-old, Caucasian male who was admitted to a residential treatment facility with presenting problems including parent–child conflict, poor peer interactions, lying, stealing, physical aggression, poor school performance, truancy, suicidal ideation, and suspected drug use.

Oliver is the only child born to his parents who were never married. His father left his mother when she was pregnant with Oliver, and he has never had any contact with his father. His mother is very resentful of having been abandoned by Oliver's father and is reported to project this resentment onto her son. Reports from previous evaluations indicate a failure on the part of Oliver's mother to bond with him. When asked, his mother cannot identify any positive qualities that Oliver has. Oliver believes that his mother sees him as a burden, and unfortunately this perception appears to be accurate.

Oliver's mother reports that he was over–active from a very young age. At the age of six, Oliver was diagnosed as having an Attention Deficit Hyper–Activity disorder after recurring problems with biting, hitting, getting out of his seat, and non–compliant behavior. He was prescribed Ritalin, which he took continuously for five years. Recently, he has refused to take this medication because he believes that it has stunted his growth (Oliver is considerably smaller than the norm for his age).

Oliver has done very poorly in school because of severe behavioral problems. This, in spite of a Full Scale IQ of 120 as measured with the WISC–R. He has been placed in Severe Behavioral Handicap classes and has refused to do his school work saying that it was too easy. He has been diagnosed as having a developmental math disorder.

Oliver has been in one mental-health treatment program or another since the age of 11. He had one psychiatric hospitalization at the age of 12 and he was diagnosed as having an Attention Deficit Hyperactivity Disorder, Oppositional Defiant Disorder, and Dysthymia. He was placed in one foster home for a period of 10 months. However, this placement was terminated at the request of the foster family who felt that they could no longer tolerate Oliver's stealing, lying, fighting, and attention–seeking behavior. He has run away from home several times, and was placed in a transitional living center before the current referral to the residential treatment facility.

Upon admission to the facility, Oliver

presented with somewhat constricted affect, grandiose and illogical thinking, and a generally defensive and guarded demeanor. He initially refused to complete any psychological testing.

Two weeks after his admission, Oliver began complaining that he believes he is "crazy," and has had thoughts like Jeffrey Dahmer for a long time. He reported experiencing very omnipotent fantasies and had difficulty carrying on a conversation. The treatment team viewed Oliver's presentation as a response to feelings of worthlessness and rejection.

Three weeks after his admission to the residential treatment facility, Oliver agreed to complete the MMPI–A.

MMPI–A INTERPRETATION
Profile Validity

Oliver responded to all the MMPI–A items. His scores on the validity scales indicate that he was able to provide a coherent and consistent set of responses to the test. Oliver produced elevated scores on scale F and its subscales F_1 and F_2. The difference between his scores on the subscales did not indicate a substantial alteration in Oliver's approach to the test between the first and second halves of the booklet.

The possibility that random responding contributed substantially to Oliver's elevated score on F is counter–indicated by his within-normal-limits score on VRIN. Clinically, Oliver was seen as presenting with increasingly unusual thought processes. His clinically observed difficulties were consistent with Oliver's level of elevation on F, indicating against over–reporting as an interpretation for his score on this scale. Oliver's scores on L and K were within normal limits.

Overall, Oliver's scores on the MMPI–A validity scales indicate that he produced a valid MMPI–A profile. He responded relevantly to the test items and reported a number of unusual experiences that are consistent with his clinical presentation. There is no indication of distorted responding in this protocol.

Current Level of Adjustment

Oliver's scores on the MMPI–A indicate that he is experiencing severe adjustment difficulties at this time. He produced a positive slope on the MMPI–A clinical scales, with most of the elevation on the right–hand side of the profile, a pattern indicative of severe psychological turmoil and confusion and the possibility that he may be experiencing psychotic symptoms. Oliver also produced a large number of highly elevated scores on several of the MMPI–A content scales, supporting further the interpretation that he was presenting with extreme dysfunction at the time of the evaluation. His elevated score on F is also consistent with this interpretation. Although his profile indicates that Oliver is likely experiencing extreme turmoil and confusion, his scores indicate that he is not reporting or experiencing a considerable amount of anxiety associated with his current level of adjustment.

Symptoms and Traits

Oliver produced a highly elevated score on Scale 9 coupled with an extremely low score on Scale 2. This pattern indicates that he is likely very restless and may be presenting with overt symptoms of a manic episode. He is likely over–active and feeling excessively energetic, he may have difficulties falling asleep, he may present with an inappropriately euphoric mood and considerable emotional lability. These scores indicate further that Oliver may present with pressured speech and flight of ideas, and that he may have a very grandiose self–view. He is likely to appear superficially very friendly and comfortable around others. Oliver is likely to act out in an impulsive manner, and may have considerable disciplinary and academic difficulties in school because of his acting-out tendencies.

Oliver's elevated score on Scale 4 provides further indication that he is prone to an externalizing pattern of behavior, that he likely tends to be aggressive to others and inconsiderate of their needs and feelings, that he tends to be resentful toward figures of authority, and that he may reject the traditional values of society. He is prone to risk–taking and sensation–seeking and, as a result, is at increased risk for developing a substance-use problem. Although he may be able to create a favorable self–impression, it is likely that he tends to be unreliable and has difficulties maintaining interpersonal relationships.

Oliver's elevated score on Scale 8 indicates that he may presently be experiencing considerable confusion and disorganization. His level of elevation on this scale indicates the possibility that he may be experiencing psychotic symptoms including delusions and hallucinations. This interpretation is supported by his pattern of scores on the subscales for Scale 8 and his elevated score on the content scale Adolescent Bizarre Mentation (A–biz). His score on this scale indicates further that in spite of a confident self–presentation, Oliver may be plagued by feelings of inferiority and self–doubt. He likely has great difficulties forming trusting relationships with others.

Oliver's elevated score on Scale 6 supports the interpretation that he tends to be very suspicious and guarded around others, that he harbors feelings of anger and resentment toward others, that he is prone to blame others for his difficulties, and that he may present as somewhat immature for his age. His pattern of scores on the subscales for this scale indicates that he may be experiencing persecutory delusions.

Oliver's scores on the MMPI–A content scales provide further information regarding his present difficulties. He produced a very elevated score on the Adolescent Conduct Problems (A–con) scale, indicating that he acknowledges extreme acting-out behavior. He reports engaging in a variety of unruly, disrespectful, and unlawful behaviors. When caught, he is likely to attempt to blame others for his actions. Oliver's extreme elevation on this scale indicates that his acknowledgment of acting-out behaviors may take on the form of bragging. Severe acting out appears presently to be an integral part of his identity.

Oliver's elevated scores on Adolescent Family Problems (A–fam) and Adolescent School Problems (A–sch) indicate that most of his acting-out behaviors may be seen in these two environments. He describes a very turbulent and non–supportive family life and likely feels distant and alienated from members of his family. He does not believe that he can turn to them for help in times of need. Oliver's acting-out behaviors are likely to cause him considerable disciplinary problems at school, and he is likely to have academic problems as well. His elevated score on Adolescent Anger (A–ang) indicates that some of Oliver's acting-out tendencies may be expressed through overt acts of aggression and hostility toward others, and that he tends generally to be irritable and short–tempered.

Oliver's elevated score on the scale A–biz indicates that he presents with a variety of psychotic symptoms that may include delusions and hallucinations. He likely feels that there is something wrong with his mind and may believe that there are others who seek to harm him. The very strong signs in Oliver's profile that he abuses alcohol and drugs (discussed later) indicate the need to examine what role these substances may play in some of the unusual symptoms he reports.

His elevated score on Adolescent Cynicism (A–cyn) is consistent with other indications in Oliver's profile that he tends to be very mistrustful and suspicious of the motives of others, particularly when they attempt to be friendly and helpful to him. Oliver likely believes that people look out only for their own interests, and he does the same.

Oliver's elevated score on Adolescent Depression (A–dep) appears, on the face of it, to be at odds with his very low score on Scale 2. A primary difference between these two scales involves the area of psychomotor functioning. Whereas Scale 2 contains a number of items that are keyed in the direction of psychomotor retardation, A–dep has very few such items. The latter scale has a greater emphasis on subjective reports of dysphoric affect and cognitions.

Examination of Oliver's scores on the subscales of Scale 2 indicates that he indeed produced a very low score on the subscale Psychomotor Retardation, a score that is consistent with other indications in his MMPI–A profile that Oliver may currently be experiencing excessive energy and stimulation. Nevertheless, his elevated score on A–dep indicates that Oliver does acknowledge some dysphoric affect along with current grandiose ideation.

Oliver's elevated score on Adolescent Health Concerns (A–hea) indicates that he complains of some physical problems at this time. His moderate level of elevation on this scale indicates that Oliver's physical concerns or complaints may be limited to one or two areas of functioning.

His highly elevated score on Adolescent Negative Treatment Indicators (A–trt) indicates that Oliver is likely very mistrusting of mental health professionals, that he may have difficulties opening up and self–disclosing to others, and that he may be ambivalent about his present need for treatment.

A final elevation of note is Oliver's score on the Immaturity (IMM) scale. His score on this scale indicates that Oliver may be developmentally immature for his age, that he may be easily frustrated and quick to anger, and that he may engage in defiant–resistant behavior.

Overall, Oliver's MMPI–A profile indicates that he is experiencing very severe problems at this time. He is very restless and over–active, and may be experiencing a manic or hypomanic episode. His speech is likely pressured and his affect may be inappropriately euphoric, he is impulsive and tends to exercise poor judgment. Oliver's MMPI–A profile indicates that he may be experiencing delusional thinking and hallucinations at this time.

In addition, Oliver's profile indicates that he is prone to extreme acting-out behavior and that he likely has problems with members of his family and at school. He has difficulties controlling his temper and may become physically aggressive toward others. Oliver may harbor deep-rooted insecurities and fears of inadequacy, which may fuel some of his acting out tendencies. Oliver may give the impression of being friendly and outgoing, but he is unlikely to form long–lasting relationships. He tends to view others as a source of threat, rather than support, and holds a generally misanthropic view of other people. Oliver is likely to be viewed by others as immature.

Diagnostic Suggestions

Oliver's MMPI–A profile raises a number of diagnostic possibilities that require further consideration and examination. There are very strong indications that he may presently be experiencing a manic or hypomanic episode, raising the possibility that Oliver may have a bipolar disorder. The possibilities of schizophrenia or a schizoaffective disorder also need to be considered. Oliver's MMPI–A profile provides very strong indications of a severe conduct disorder as well.

Oliver produced highly elevated scores on all three MMPI–A substance-abuse scales. His elevation on the Revised MacAndrew scale (MAC–R) is consistent with other indications in his profile that Oliver is inclined toward sensation-seeking and risk–taking, and that these proclivities place him at substantial risk for developing a drug and/or alcohol problem. His elevated score on the Alcohol/Drug Problem Proneness (PRO) scale provides further evidences of Oliver's increased risk for problems in this area and indicates that he may be susceptible to the negative influences of peers who may be involved with drugs and/or alcohol. His highly elevated score on the Alcohol/Drug Problem Acknowledgment (ACK) scale, indicates that Oliver admits excessive and problematic use of alcohol and drugs.

Treatment Recommendations

Strong indications that Oliver may be experiencing a manic episode accompanied by psychotic symptoms suggest the desirability of an immediate referral for a psychiatric evaluation to determine his need for psychotropic medication. Once his condition is stabilized, the focus of treatment may shift to Oliver's extreme acting-out behaviors. There are indications in this profile that his acting-out tendencies may represent a means for Oliver to cover up feelings of inferiority and social inadequacy. In light of the background information in this case, such feelings are certainly to be expected. Thus, in devising an intervention strategy for Oliver, it may be desirable to combine a highly structured behavioral management program with individual therapy designed to assist Oliver in identifying and confronting his feelings of inadequacy. Further evaluation of Oliver's pattern of alcohol and/or drug use is also indicated.

Oliver's elevated score on A–trt indicates that his therapist will face considerable challenges in attempting to develop a therapeutic relationship. However, this score is most effectively viewed as an indication of challenge rather than as a cause for pessimism.

OUTCOME

One day after completing the MMPI–A Oliver was interviewed once more with the goal of determining a diagnosis. During this interview he presented with extreme restlessness and agitation, markedly pressured speech, very euphoric mood, and very disorganized thinking. Oliver described grandiose delusional beliefs as well as considerable fears that peers and members of the staff were jealous of him and might try to harm him. He was diagnosed as having a bipolar disorder in a manic phase with psychotic features as well as a severe conduct disorder. Further evaluation of his substance-use pattern indicated a Polysubstance Abuse diagnosis.

Oliver was referred for a psychiatric examination to determine appropriate medication. The examining psychiatrist concurred with the psychologist's diagnosis and prescribed Lithium. Oliver initially resisted medication, but eventually, after being transferred to a secured unit, he consented and began taking the prescribed medication. He responded well to the treatment and his manic episode was viewed as being in full remission after three weeks.

Following stabilization with medication, Oliver was transferred back to an open residential unit where a behavioral management program was instituted along with intensive individual psychotherapy.

MMPI-A*

Extended Score Report

ID Number 15

Oliver

Male

Age 14

7/02/93

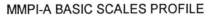

MMPI-A BASIC SCALES PROFILE

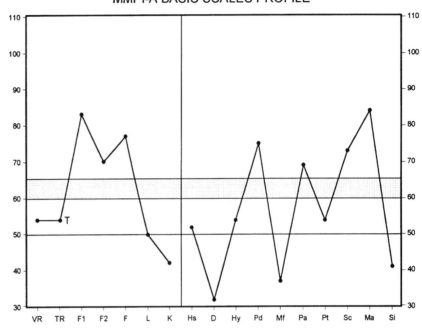

	VR	TR	F1	F2	F	L	K	Hs	D	Hy	Pd	Mf	Pa	Pt	Sc	Ma	Si
Raw Score:	6	10	17	15	32	3	9	9	9	23	31	16	20	22	42	34	19
T-Score:	54	54	83	70	77	50	42	52	32	54	75	37	69	54	73	84	41

Response %:   100   100   100   100   100   100   100   100   100   100   100   100   100   100   100   100   100

Cannot Say (Raw) =   0   Percent True: 65   Percent False: 35

Welsh Code: 9"48'6+-371/0:52# F'+-L/K:

CASE 15
"OLIVER"

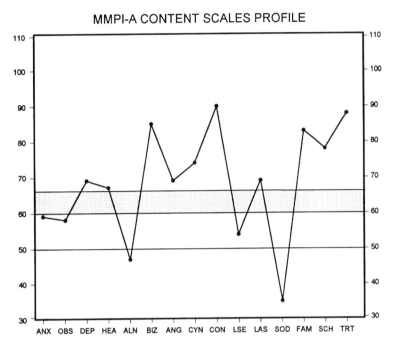

MMPI-A CONTENT SCALES PROFILE

	ANX	OBS	DEP	HEA	ALN	BIZ	ANG	CYN	CON	LSE	LAS	SOD	FAM	SCH	TRT
Raw Score:	12	10	16	17	5	14	13	20	22	7	10	1	26	14	21
T-Score:	59	58	69	67	47	85	69	74	90	54	69	35	83	78	88
Response %:	100	100	100	100	100	100	100	100	100	100	100	100	100	100	100

SUPPLEMENTARY SCORE REPORT

	Raw Score	T Score	Resp %
MacAndrew Alcoholism-Revised (MAC-R)	34	79	100
Alcohol/Drug Problem Acknowledgement (ACK)	11	79	100
Alcohol/Drug Problem Proneness (PRO)	30	80	100
Immaturity Scale (IMM)	27	72	100
Anxiety (A)	21	59	100
Repression (R)	11	44	100

Depression Subscales (Harris-Lingoes)

	Raw Score	T Score	Resp %
Subjective Depression (D1)	7	46	100
Psychomotor Retardation (D2)	2	36	100
Physical Malfunctioning (D3)	1	35	100
Mental Dullness (D4)	3	47	100
Brooding (D5)	4	56	100

Hysteria Subscales (Harris-Lingoes)

	Raw Score	T Score	Resp %
Denial of Social Anxiety (Hy1)	4	55	100
Need for Affection (Hy2)	4	46	100
Lassitude-Malaise (Hy3)	4	50	100
Somatic Complaints (Hy4)	7	60	100
Inhibition of Aggression (Hy5)	4	59	100

Psychopathic Deviate Subscales (Harris-Lingoes)

	Raw Score	T Score	Resp %
Familial Discord (Pd1)	6	64	100
Authority Problems (Pd2)	7	73	100
Social Imperturbability (Pd3)	5	61	100
Social Alienation (Pd4)	6	55	100
Self-Alienation (Pd5)	9	69	100

Paranoia Subscales (Harris-Lingoes)

	Raw Score	T Score	Resp %
Persecutory Ideas (Pa1)	10	71	100
Poignancy (Pa2)	4	55	100
Naivete (Pa3)	1	34	100

Schizophrenia Subscales (Harris-Lingoes)

Social Alienation (Sc1)	8	56	100
Emotional Alienation (Sc2)	5	65	100
Lack of Ego Mastery, Cognitive (Sc3)	7	68	100
Lack of Ego Mastery, Conative (Sc4)	9	69	100
Lack of Ego Mastery, Defective Inhibition (Sc5)	6	62	100
Bizarre Sensory Experiences (Sc6)	13	74	100

Hypomania Subscales (Harris-Lingoes)

Amorality (Ma1)	6	73	100
Psychomotor Acceleration (Ma2)	9	62	100
Imperturbability (Ma3)	6	68	100
Ego Inflation (Ma4)	6	58	100

Social Introversion Subscales (Ben-Porath, Hostetler, Butcher, & Graham)

Shyness / Self-Consciousness (Si1)	2	36	100
Social Avoidance (Si2)	0	38	100
Alienation--Self and Others (Si3)	11	60	100

Uniform T scores are used for Hs, D, Hy, Pd, Pa, Pt, Sc, Ma, and the Content Scales; all other MMPI-A scales use linear T scores.

End of Report

SUGGESTED ITEMS FOR FOLLOW-UP

ALCOHOL/DRUG PROBLEMS

144. I have a problem with alcohol or drugs. (T)

247. I have used alcohol excessively. (T)

342. I can express my true feelings only when I drink. (T)

458. I sometimes get into fights when drinking. (T)

467. I enjoy using marijuana. (T)

474. People often tell me I have a problem with drinking too much. (T)

FAMILY PROBLEMS

366. I have gotten many beatings. (T)

440. I have spent nights away from home when my parents did not know where I was. (T)

460. I have never run away from home. (F)

CASE 16
"PAULA"

A "NEGLECTED" TEEN

BACKGROUND

Paula is a 16-year-old, Caucasian female tested on a secured unit of a residential treatment facility. She had been at the facility for three months at the time of testing. Her presenting problems upon admission to the facility were depressive symptoms, a recent suicidal gesture, severe familial discord, chronic school problems, explosive behavior, and lower than age-appropriate self–care skills.

Paula is the older of two children born to her parents and she was raised by both parents. Her father is described as very domineering and over–involved in Paula's life. He wanted to "mandate" her treatment and was described by Paula's therapist as the most controlling parent she had ever encountered.

Paula was an only child until the age of 14 when her younger sister was born. Up until then, she was very over–protected and was treated as though she were considerably younger than her years. For example, her parents continued to take care of her grooming needs until her sister's birth. However, little attention was paid to Paula after the birth of her younger sister, and that is when her problems began.

Paula responded initially by acting out in

school where, up until her sister's birth, she had been an average student and had no disciplinary problems. She began to act out in class, was very disrespectful toward her teachers, and was suspended from school for several days. At home, she made a rather serious suicide attempt and was hospitalized in a child and adolescent psychiatric unit of a general hospital. She was eventually released, but continued to be very depressed and was subsequently re–hospitalized twice following suicidal threats.

Following her third hospitalization, an attempt was made to place Paula in a therapeutic foster home. Although they ostensibly agreed to this placement, her parents, particularly Paula's father, interfered with her treatment and she was eventually returned to their home.

Three months before the present evaluation, Paula made another suicidal gesture and was placed in a secure unit of a residential treatment facility. Initially, she declined to complete any psychological tests. Her behavior on the unit was viewed as manipulative and destructive, and she had very poor relationships with her peers. She became the unit's "scapegoat" and was unable to make any friends. She made several unauthorized attempts to leave the facility.

One month after her admission Paula was prescribed anti–depressant medication which she agreed to ingest. Within several weeks, her mood improved and she became more active on the unit. However, she continued to have very poor social relationships. She agreed to take the MMPI–A after her therapist suggested that this might help with her treatment.

MMPI–A INTERPRETATION
Profile Validity

Paula produced a valid MMPI–A profile, but she failed to respond to a relatively large number of items (13). Examination of the list of Omitted Items indicates a number of themes in the content of the items she refused to answer. Several items deal with depressed mood and several others deal with dependency issues. Although Paula's failure to respond to these items cannot, in itself, be interpreted as meaning that she has problems in these areas, it does indicate a reluctance on her part to discuss these issues at this time. The number of omitted items is insufficient to raise questions about the validity of the entire profile and the list indicates that the omitted items were dispersed throughout the test. Examination of the percentage of items answered on a scale-by-scale basis indicates that Paula responded to 90% or more of all the full scales, although several subscale scores (Hy$_3$, Sc$_3$, Sc$_4$, and Ma$_1$) are based on fewer than 90% of their items and should therefore not be interpreted.

Examination of Paula's scores on the remaining validity scales indicates that she provided consistent and coherent responses and did not approach the test with a response set. Her scores on these scales are all within normal limits and thus indicate that she produced a valid and interpretable MMPI–A profile.

Current Level of Adjustment

Paula's MMPI–A profile indicates that she reports moderate adjustment problems at this time. She produced elevated scores on several of the clinical scales. However, her most prominent elevation is on a scale related primarily to acting-out problems rather than to anxiety or distress. A similar pattern is found on her content scale scores. Overall, her scores on the MMPI–A indicate that Paula is reporting having some psychological problems at this time. However, she does not appear to be experiencing a considerable amount of distress as a result of these problems.

Symptoms and Traits

Paula's highest elevation on the MMPI–A clinical scale profile is on Scale 4. This indicates that she probably presents with a variety of acting–out problems, is likely to resent and get into conflicts with authority figures and with members of her family, may have a tendency toward alcohol and/or drug-use problems, and that she is likely to be impulsive and may also be aggressive. Her score on this scale suggests further that Paula tends to be self–centered, and she may not accept responsibility for her problems.

Paula produced secondary elevation on clinical Scale 6. Her score on this scale suggests that Paula tends to be guarded and suspicious of others, she may view others as a source of threat, rather than support, she may be inclined to project blame for her difficulties onto others, and she may believe that others seek to do her harm. She may be overly sensitive to criticism and likely views the world as hostile and rejecting.

Paula also produced mild, but clinically significant elevations on clinical scales 2 and 7. These scores indicate that Paula reports experiencing some symptoms of depression and anxiety at this time but presently is not overwhelmed by these difficulties.

Paula's most elevated score on the MMPI–A content scales is on Adolescent School Problems (A–sch). This indicates that she reports having many difficulties at school and that she likely has both academic and disciplinary problems. She very likely dislikes school and views it as a threatening environment. Her acting-out tendencies appear to be expressed most notably in the school setting.

Paula also produced a highly elevated score on Adolescent Anger (A–ang), indicating that she acknowledges having anger-control problems. She may become destructive when she is angry and may generally feel irritable and impatient with others. She may throw temper tantrums if she does not get her own way.

Paula's score on the Adolescent Family Problems (A–fam) scale is also elevated. This score indicates that she reports considerable turmoil and conflict in her family, most notably between herself and her parents. She may believe that she cannot count on her family in times of need. She may be searching for ways to disengage from them.

Paula also produced an elevated score on Adolescent Anxiety (A–anx), indicating that she does report experiencing some subjective symptoms of anxiety at this time. In contrast, her score on Adolescent Depression (A–dep) falls below the clinical cutoff. This pattern would suggest that Paula's elevations on clinical scales 2 and 7 stem primarily from her experience of anxiety rather than of depression.

Her elevated score on Adolescent Conduct Problems (A–con) indicates that Paula acknowledges engaging in some anti–social acting–out behaviors. However, her level of elevation on this scale is considerably lower than on some of the other content scales. This indicates that much of the elevation on clinical Scale 4 may be attributable to school- and family-related acting-out problems rather than to a more generalized tendency toward rule breaking.

Finally, Paula produced marginally elevated scores on Adolescent Low Self–Esteem (A–lse) and Adolescent Low Aspirations (A–las). These scores indicate that Paula tends to hold a negative self–view, that she may have very low expectations for success and, as a result, she does not strive very hard to succeed.

Overall, Paula's MMPI-A profile indicates that she has substantial behavioral control problems at this time. She tends to be angry and resentful, and she is most likely to express these feelings in a negative manner in school and in her relationships with members of her family. She views her family as a source of turmoil and conflict rather than of support. She tends generally to be guarded and suspicious of others. However, she is not particularly uncomfortable in social relationships. In fact, she may be capable of generating a positive self–impression. Nevertheless, Paula's anger-control problems are likely to bring about conflict in interpersonal relationships. In school, she likely has both academic and disciplinary problems. Paula tends to have a rather negative self–view, and, as a result, she may have given up hope of improving her situation. She is experiencing some anxiety at this time, but her level of distress is somewhat lower than would be expected given the circumstances of this evaluation.

Diagnostic Suggestions

Paula's MMPI–A profile suggests a strong likelihood of a conduct disorder. In addition, her elevated score on Scale 4 coupled with her elevated score on the Alcohol/Drug Problem Proneness (PRO) scale suggests that she is at risk for developing an alcohol or drug problem. Although these scores do not indicate the presence of such a problem at this time, they do suggest that Paula may be susceptible to the negative influences of peers who may use these substances. The indication in her profile that Paula does not tend to be uncomfortable in social situations suggests that she is likely capable of forming social relationships and her generally negativistic attitude may indeed lead her to interact with negative peers.

There also are indications in Paula's MMPI–A profile that she has considerable anger problems, that she experiences some emotional lability, and that she has poor self–esteem. Consequently, the possibility of an emerging personality disorder, possibly with borderline features, should be considered.

Treatment Recommendations

Paula's MMPI–A profile indicates the

need for assistance in behavioral management. It appears that anti–depressant medication has alleviated most of her mood symptoms, but she continues to exhibit considerable acting-out problems. A contingency–based behavioral management program may be beneficial to assist in controlling Paula's acting–out and anger control problems. Also, individual therapy may be indicated to help Paula build her self–esteem, and family therapy is indicated to assist Paula and her family in dealing with the considerable turmoil in their family life at this time. Paula's relatively low score on the content scale Negative Treatment Indicators (A–trt) may be viewed as a positive indication that she presently may be open to therapeutic intervention.

OUTCOME

Following her assessment, Paula's therapist provided her with feedback regarding her MMPI–A profile. The feedback consisted mostly of the descriptive information included in this interpretation. However, it was presented in a supportive, nonthreatening manner. She continued to make progress in individual therapy and, with the aid of a behavioral control program, began to manage the expression of her anger in a much more adaptive manner. Her performance in the facility's school improved to her level of academic achievements before the onset of her difficulties.

Unfortunately, attempts to engage Paula's family in her treatment were unsuccessful. Her father refused to participate in family therapy sessions and her mother stated that, because she cannot drive, she could not come to the facility without Paula's father. Her father eventually withdrew Paula from the facility, and she stopped attending outpatient therapy sessions within a month of leaving the facility.

MMPI-A*

Extended Score Report

.

ID Number 16

Paula

Female

Age 16

2/11/93

MMPI-A BASIC SCALES PROFILE

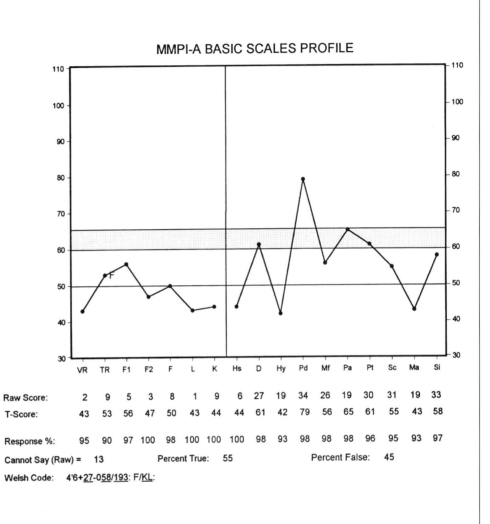

	VR	TR	F1	F2	F	L	K	Hs	D	Hy	Pd	Mf	Pa	Pt	Sc	Ma	Si
Raw Score:	2	9	5	3	8	1	9	6	27	19	34	26	19	30	31	19	33
T-Score:	43	53	56	47	50	43	44	44	61	42	79	56	65	61	55	43	58
Response %:	95	90	97	100	98	100	100	100	98	93	98	98	98	96	95	93	97

Cannot Say (Raw) = 13   Percent True: 55   Percent False: 45

Welsh Code: 4'6+27-058/193: F/KL:

CASE 16
"PAULA"

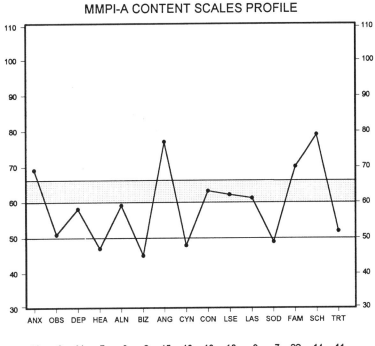

MMPI-A CONTENT SCALES PROFILE

	ANX	OBS	DEP	HEA	ALN	BIZ	ANG	CYN	CON	LSE	LAS	SOD	FAM	SCH	TRT
Raw Score:	16	9	14	7	9	2	15	13	13	10	9	7	22	14	11
T-Score:	69	51	58	47	59	45	77	48	63	62	61	49	70	79	52
Response %:	100	93	92	100	95	89	100	91	96	94	100	100	100	100	100

SUPPLEMENTARY SCORE REPORT

	Raw Score	T Score	Resp %
MacAndrew Alcoholism-Revised (MAC-R)	22	55	98
Alcohol/Drug Problem Acknowledgement (ACK)	5	56	100
Alcohol/Drug Problem Proneness (PRO)	27	75	100
Immaturity Scale (IMM)	20	63	98
Anxiety (A)	24	59	91
Repression (R)	12	46	100

Depression Subscales (Harris-Lingoes)

Subjective Depression (D1)	16	63	97
Psychomotor Retardation (D2)	6	57	100
Physical Malfunctioning (D3)	4	52	100
Mental Dullness (D4)	7	62	100
Brooding (D5)	6	60	90

Hysteria Subscales (Harris-Lingoes)

Denial of Social Anxiety (Hy1)	2	43	100
Need for Affection (Hy2)	3	42	92
Lassitude-Malaise (Hy3)	6	55	87
Somatic Complaints (Hy4)	5	50	100
Inhibition of Aggression (Hy5)	1	35	100

Psychopathic Deviate Subscales (Harris-Lingoes)

Familial Discord (Pd1)	5	56	100
Authority Problems (Pd2)	5	65	100
Social Imperturbability (Pd3)	2	43	100
Social Alienation (Pd4)	10	71	100
Self-Alienation (Pd5)	9	67	92

Paranoia Subscales (Harris-Lingoes)

Persecutory Ideas (Pa1)	9	68	100
Poignancy (Pa2)	6	62	100
Naivete (Pa3)	3	46	100

Schizophrenia Subscales (Harris-Lingoes)

Social Alienation (Sc1)	11	64	100
Emotional Alienation (Sc2)	3	54	91
Lack of Ego Mastery, Cognitive (Sc3)	2	45	70
Lack of Ego Mastery, Conative (Sc4)	7	60	86
Lack of Ego Mastery, Defective Inhibition (Sc5)	6	58	100
Bizarre Sensory Experiences (Sc6)	2	40	95

Hypomania Subscales (Harris-Lingoes)

Amorality (Ma1)	1	39	83
Psychomotor Acceleration (Ma2)	6	44	91
Imperturbability (Ma3)	3	50	100
Ego Inflation (Ma4)	4	47	100

Social Introversion Subscales (Ben-Porath, Hostetler, Butcher, & Graham)

Shyness / Self-Consciousness (Si1)	7	52	100
Social Avoidance (Si2)	1	45	100
Alienation--Self and Others (Si3)	13	63	94

Uniform T scores are used for Hs, D, Hy, Pd, Pa, Pt, Sc, Ma, and the Content Scales; all other
MMPI-A scales use linear T scores.

OMITTED ITEMS

The following items were omitted by the client. It may be helpful to discuss these item omissions with this individual to determine the reason for non-compliance with test instructions.

62. Most of the time I feel blue.
83. I have met problems so full of possibilities that I have been unable to make up my mind about them.
84. I believe women ought to have as much sexual freedom as men.
91. I am happy most of the time.
118. I often wonder what hidden reason another person may have for doing something nice for me.
173. There is something wrong with my mind.
183. In walking I am very careful to step over sidewalk cracks.
234. At times I have been so entertained by the cleverness of some criminals that I have hoped they would get away with it.
280. I am apt to pass up something I want to do when others feel that it isn't worth doing.
291. I often feel as if things are not real.
305. I have more trouble concentrating than others seem to have.
330. People generally demand more respect for their own rights than they are willing to allow for others.
448. Most people think they can depend on me.

End of Report

SUGGESTED ITEMS FOR FOLLOW-UP

None

CONCLUDING REMARKS

It is our hope that the 16 cases presented in this book illustrate the richness of information that is contained in an adolescent's MMPI–A profile. We have sought to demonstrate the breadth and depth of data that may be gleaned with appropriate and sophisticated use of the test. We have also, wherever possible, incorporated information from other psychometric instruments. Our purpose in doing so was to emphasize that the MMPI–A is but one of several tests that can and should be used to assess adolescent functioning and behavior.

The MMPI–A profiles interpreted in this book illustrate two important contributions that the test can make in a variety of clinical settings and assessment contexts. First, the test provides a cost–effective vehicle for obtaining a large amount of clinically useful information. In all 16 cases there was substantial congruence between the extensive background and outcome information available and the interpretations suggested by the MMPI–A profile. This congruence provides a tangible illustration of the validity of the MMPI–A as a measure of behavioral and emotional functioning of adolescents.

A second contribution, demonstrated in several of the cases, is the ability of the MMPI–A to alert the clinician to important issues that have yet to surface. The most dramatic example of the MMPI–A providing clinical staff with important and as yet undetected aspects of an adolescent's functioning is seen in Case 11, the case of "Kyle," who manifested severe psychotic decompensation which was predicted by an MMPI–A that he had just completed. Having such an early warning allowed staff to respond quickly and appropriately to a crisis situation. Similar examples are found in several other cases in this book.

In closing, we would like to express once more our appreciation and respect for the youngsters whose cases were discussed and analyzed in this book. All of them knew, when they completed the instrument, that their test scores might be used for research and educational purposes. We are indebted to them for their cooperation. We hope that our collaborative efforts as test–takers and test–interpreters will benefit other youngsters who turn or are referred to mental-health professionals for assistance.

INDEX